Acclaim for

my caesare

~

"The C-section experience is as varied as life itself—there's guilt
and gratitude, pride and regret. These mothers illuminate the whole
spectrum with depth, urgency, and humor. *My Caesarean* is the
antidote to alienation, and I dearly wish I'd had it before my own
births. I'm so glad we have it now."—**MEAGHAN O'CONNELL,**
author of *And Now We Have Everything*

"A fresh and compelling range of voices lifting a painful
topic into the light."—**KATHLEEN GLASGOW,**
New York Times–bestselling author of *Girl in Pieces*

"The essays in *My Caesarean* refuse to idealize the birth
experience and show it in all its stunning unexpectedness. This
is a beautiful and important book that should be prominently
shelved in the birth and parenting section of every bookstore."
—**JULIE SCHUMACHER,** award-winning author of
Dear Committee Members and *The Shakespeare Requirement*

"This collection gathers the overlooked and under-processed
experiences of C-sections—each importantly different, each
importantly the same—and prompts robust reflection. Together these
voices create a much-needed community that will comfort and
challenge, enlighten and affirm."—**BETH ANN FENNELLY,**
poet laureate of Mississippi and author of *Great with Child*

my
caesarean

Twenty-One Mothers on the
C-Section Experience and After

WITHDRAWN

Edited by Amanda Fields
and Rachel Moritz

THE EXPERIMENT

NEW YORK

The Experiment, LLC, 220 East 23rd Street, Suite 600, New York, NY 10010-4658
theexperimentpublishing.com

This book contains the opinions and ideas of its authors. It is intended to provide helpful and informative material on the subjects addressed in the book. It is sold with the understanding that the authors and publisher are not engaged in rendering medical, health, or any other kind of personal professional services in the book. The authors and publisher specifically disclaim all responsibility for any liability, loss, or risk—personal or otherwise—that is incurred as a consequence, directly or indirectly, of the use and application of any of the contents of this book.

Many of the designations used by manufacturers and sellers to distinguish their products are claimed as trademarks. Where those designations appear in this book and The Experiment was aware of a trademark claim, the designations have been capitalized.

The Experiment's books are available at special discounts when purchased in bulk for premiums and sales promotions as well as for fund-raising or educational use. For details, contact us at info@ theexperimentpublishing.com.

Library of Congress Cataloging-in-Publication Data

Names: Fields, Amanda, editor. | Moritz, Rachel, editor.
Title: My caesarean : twenty-one mothers on the C-section experience and
    after / edited by Amanda Fields and Rachel Moritz.
Description: New York : The Experiment, LLC, [2019] | Includes
    bibliographical references.
Identifiers: LCCN 2019004739 (print) | LCCN 2019009376 (ebook) | ISBN
    9781615195534 (ebook) | ISBN 9781615195527 (pbk.)
Subjects: LCSH: Cesarean section. | Short stories.
Classification: LCC RG761 (ebook) | LCC RG761 .M9 2019 (print) | DDC
    618.8/6--dc23
LC record available at https://lccn.loc.gov/2019004739

ISBN 978-1-61519-552-7
Ebook ISBN 978-1-61519-553-4

Cover design by Sarah Smith | Text design by Sarah Schneider
Author photographs by John Lovretta (Amanda Fields) and Maya Washington (Rachel Moritz)

Manufactured in the United States of America
First printing May 2019
10 9 8 7 6 5 4 3 2 1

For C-section mothers and their families

Contents

Stitches

Twice they opened me
and twice, after sewing me shut,

    they said the thread would dissolve,

    they said my body would dissolve

the thread. But see how frugal
I've become, saving every stitch

    for future alterations and repairs.

    Any woman with my blood

saves—is a saver. When given one
sheet of paper, my daughter

    cuts out the heart she wants

    and keeps the scraps for stars,

snowflakes, flowers. Twice
they cut babies from my body,

    but the body remains.

    See how nothing is wasted.

The more they cut, the more I have.

—Maggie Smith

Foreword

Maggie Smith

HOW MANY YEARS DID it take me to write about my own caesareans? Too many. My children were born in 2008 and 2012, and my poem "Stitches," first published in *Linebreak*, appeared in my third book, *Good Bones*, in 2017. Regardless of how long it took me to come to this poem, it's taught me about myself, about how I actually feel about my birth experiences. And hearing from readers that this poem resonates with them, and that their own experience is reflected in mine, has meant so much to me. This combination of insight and resonance is what I hope readers find in *My Caesarean*.

Our children's births are individual, but these essays have opened my eyes to the caesarean experience as a shared experience. The anthology includes diverse perspectives, from emergency to elective C-sections, from traumatic experiences to empowering ones. In "I Didn't Dream of Pregnancy," Tyrese Coleman writes about choosing a caesarean as a way of reclaiming the body, and the vagina in particular, after sexual trauma: "Forgive me for not wanting to associate my children with the continued violation of my body." As SooJin Pate writes, "I wanted my daughter to come through me—not to be plucked out from some man-made surgical incision. This process of coming through me was especially significant because of my history as a transracial adoptee." These complexities are what make this anthology essential reading.

My own experience is not unusual. My firstborn daughter was face-up and resisted the midwife's and OB's attempts to turn her. I labored for almost twenty-four hours. I remember vividly getting on my hands and knees near the end to push, but I have no idea how, with an epidural in place, I was able to do it. Had I imagined it wrong? How could I have moved myself into that position if I had been numb from the waist down? But I did.

Catherine Newman narrates a similar experience with pushing on her hands and knees while numb. Her account helped me trust myself regardless of how seemingly impossible my account was. Yes, it happened that way. Yes. I was there. Newman also describes the labor as "a strobe-lit horror-movie" and a "rave, the kind that goes blurry and death-defying after someone slips you a roofie." *Yes!* I thought—or perhaps even said aloud in the room—as I read this. Yes, this is what it was like for me. When the epidural ran dry and the anesthesiologist was in an emergency C-section and was not available to help me, I wanted to jump out the plate glass window of my birthing suite just to feel something other than my intense contractions. Even another kind of pain. Even obliteration.

Eventually, it became clear to the doctor and midwife that my baby was not going to budge. *She has always done things her way*, we joke now, *and that started in the womb*. I knew, when my daughter was essentially stuck inside me, that there was no other way. Even so, I was disappointed. This disappointment is not universal but it is common. With my first child, I remember crying, feeling defeated, feeling as if I'd failed at something natural and instinctual— something I was supposed to be able to do. I wanted the pain to end, and I wanted her out in the world, but I was not prepared for the fear I'd feel in the operating room. Jacinda Townsend writes, "After twenty-seven hours of labor, I'd been slit open like a hog." *Yes!* I thought. My organs had been unpacked from my abdomen, for god's sake! I know this because the midwife borrowed my husband's camera when we went into surgery, and took photographs. Now I can show my daughter her birth: *There you are, and there are Mommy's intestines!*

As LaToya Jordan writes, "I don't think I was put back together correctly. . . . I was rearranged as a mother. I'm not sure I'll ever be put back together the right way." I had been unpacked, re-assembled, cauterized, stitched, and stapled. There were so many gloved hands. I imagined myself being made on an assembly line, like a car—so many robotic arms working over me, so many tools. Amanda Fields writes of the "dull pulls and tugs from behind the curtain. . . . Then she was across the room, squalling. Then she was gone." This "vanishing act" Fields describes dovetails with some of what Rachel Moritz recounts in her essay: "I never saw our placenta or umbilical cord, two features of my pregnant body that felt like ghost children themselves. They had been packaged and sent to a medical closet in the bowels of the hospital." These feelings of separation and emptiness come up again and again in these essays and in the stories my friends and I tell about our caesareans—mother and child are separated, each helpless, each at the mercy of strangers.

If I felt alone in grieving the less-than-ideal birth of a healthy baby girl, I see here that I am not alone. Spending time with these women's words makes me feel part of a community. We have scars in common—ones we can see, yes, and perhaps others that are not visible. As Robin Schoenthaler writes, "this C-section scar saved my life. It's not a wound—it's a life door. . . . A C-section for us meant life. His life. My life." Rumi: "The wound is the place where light enters you." I see my scar daily, hard and dark from being a door between my body and the world, not once but twice, and think about what it's brought me.

Yes, both of my children were born via caesarean. Nearly four years, and two miscarriages, after the birth of my daughter, I delivered my son via a scheduled C-section. As the midwives told me, I was not a good candidate for a VBAC, given the size of my first child and the likelihood that a boy would be larger. When my son was born a week early at almost ten pounds, I admit I was relieved not to have labored with him. But the surgery wasn't less scary the second time around. I remember hearing my irregular heartbeat on the monitor in the room—I have dealt with arrhythmia on and off for years—and I thought I was dying. I started to hyperventilate; my hands went numb. I remember a lot of faces over me, talking to me, trying to keep me present and calm.

The recovery, too, was longer and more complicated with my son. Like many of the women included in this anthology, I did not feel ready to leave the hospital when my insurance company required me to leave. I remember how absurd it felt to leave the hospital after being unpacked and reassembled, and to be expected to manage around-the-clock care for a helpless newborn and a three-year-old. I was unable to climb stairs, drive, or even lift anything heavier than a jug of milk. I did not want my daughter on my tender lap. I could not take her up to bed. I couldn't carry the car seat. Meanwhile, I was up at all hours with a colicky baby, unable to rest and recuperate. I experienced postpartum anxiety and depression for the second time, as well. As Alicia Jo Rabins writes, "How strange when joy and trauma are wrapped up in each other. Is this motherhood?" In my experience, it was. And in some ways still is.

We bring some of the pain and trauma upon ourselves and upon other women, particularly when judgment enters the equation.

Sara Bates writes about the mommy wars—the passive-aggressive (and sometimes outright aggressive) shaming that happens between mothers. As Bates writes, "It took me just over a year to fully understand that my son's birth was not a test I needed to pass, not something I needed to do a certain way in order to become a worthy mother, not something to be defended or explained away or something I had to prove to anyone, or to myself."

These essays are sometimes funny, sometimes devastating, but always candid, insightful, and well-crafted. Reading *My Caesarean*, I laughed, I cried, and I may have muttered *hell yes* more than once. This book opened my eyes to other facets of the experience. One realization I had is that my children's birth experiences aren't mine alone to claim—they're also hers and his. They're ours. Of course! The narrative of their birth can't be all about my disappointment or grief, or even my joy and relief. I remember going to a job interview pregnant, carrying my daughter with me into that conference room and feeling comforted by the fact that I was not alone. I remember all the things my kids and I did together before they were born, when we shared my body.

What I've found in *My Caesarean* is a feeling—no, a deep knowing—that I am not alone. I've found a sense of community and connection with these other writer-mothers. We have similar scars but also shared gratitude, shared joy. What a gift.

MAGGIE SMITH is an award-winning poet, editor, and writer; the author of *Good Bones*, *The Well Speaks of Its Own Poison*, and *Lamp of the Body*.

Editors' Note

WHILE THE ESSAYS IN this book can't cover the range of stories that need to be told, we're here, with this collection, to begin a conversation about caesarean birth. Those of us who've brought children into the world this way have had wildly different experiences and reactions. For some, the caesarean is welcomed as a choice or necessity. Others carry ambivalence or trauma about the surgery. A new mother is often told to focus on the outcome of a healthy baby and given little information about her own physical recovery.

As C-section mothers ourselves, we were struck by the lack of time and space we had to process our surgeries, and, later, by the surprising dearth of stories we found about this common experience. We felt alone.

But, of course, we weren't. Our collaboration started with a social media thread. Rachel shared a video on Facebook showing a "natural" caesarean in the United Kingdom. This C-section was performed without a surgical drape, so the mother could watch her child being pulled from her uterus, could even reach down and touch the baby, then hold him skin-to-skin. Several women commented on the post, recounting difficult or unresolved moments from their caesareans.

Many of us had questions. What would giving birth have been like, we asked, if our C-sections hadn't been clouded with fear or emergency, covered up so we couldn't actively participate? What if we'd been given clearer information about the realities of our bodies, in some cases for months or years after, as we healed from major surgery? Had we "given birth" or passively allowed the medical world to pull babies from our bodies? And what was it like for women who scheduled caesareans or experienced few if any complications? Where were the stories of individuals who were happy with their C-sections, of women who healed quickly or didn't get caught up in these questions? Why, in pregnancy literature, was the C-section experience relegated to one chapter?

We continued the conversation outside of social media and soon realized that we had few models for processing our children's births. Most of what we had read about C-sections covered only the first six weeks postpartum. There was almost nothing out there to help us understand the experience as an embodied imprint. So we decided to draft essays about our caesareans. And while it's an overused idea, perhaps—writing as healing   the chance to share these essays, for us, was a balm. We knew there were others who needed this, too.

We're here, with this collection, because we want to hear more C-section stories.

We're here because we didn't know how or whether to resolve the complicated feelings we had about a procedure that brought our children to us. We needed to hear that some of us rejoice, and some of us don't exactly rejoice. We're here because we want to listen to the nuances of C-section birth. We're here because we haven't seen a collection devoted entirely to caesareans, and because it heartened us, when we received an outpouring of submissions, to know that other women need this, too. In editing these essays, we became immersed in the power of many voices assembled together, and the way they hold this subject up to the light. This book is here to widen our conversation about birth. We hope you will join us.

AMANDA FIELDS AND RACHEL MORITZ
May 2019

PART ONE

Birth Matters

Many who've given birth by caesarean recall a collage of images, sounds, and sensations. A blue surgical drape. A sterilized room. Numbness in the lower half of the body. Arms pinned out. The belly: pulled, stretched. Uncontrollable shaking. A baby's cry puncturing the air. And, before and after the surgery, words that describe, rationalize, evaluate. Planned. Unplanned. Convenient. Necessity. Relief. Emergency. Natural. Unnatural. Strong. Weak. Happy words. Tragic words. Words that resonate in-between.

The caesarean was once an eleventh-hour effort to save a baby. Today, one in five women around the world gives birth by C-section, with a global increase of 12.4 percent since 1990. In the Dominican Republic, Brazil, China, and Turkey, 46 to 57 percent of women give birth by caesarean. In countries such as the United States, Sri Lanka, Germany, and Albania, the rate ranges from 30 to 45 percent.[1] A variety of factors influence these rates, including approaches to medical and maternal care.

While a C-section can mean the difference between life and death, it has also become a potent symbol of contemporary childbirth. For many, it reflects the over-medicalization of labor, a process that can be dictated by hospital timelines and risk-tolerance equations. If a C-section is elective and chosen by the mother, it may be interpreted as a sign of weakness. These ideas aren't new, but they hold their grip. And when it comes to the health of women and newborns, critical issues are at play. In the US, preventable complications and maternal mortality rates, especially for Black women and trans individuals, are on the rise.[2] Those who give birth by caesarean face increased risk of infection and hemorrhage;

they're also more likely to encounter infertility and complications with future pregnancies. Caesareans can cause problems for babies, too, such as breathing difficulties that need treatment in a neonatal intensive care unit (NICU).[3]

The essays that begin this collection explore the complexities of giving birth by C-section. They speak to the necessity of the surgery for some women, as well as the disappointment or sense of failure experienced by others who felt they may not have had a say. They shed light on the range of intense emotions that accompany childbirth, and they insist that our conversations about C-section birth hold both sides of the equation: The outcome of a healthy baby matters beyond measure, *and* the way we bring children into the world is always worthy of reflection.

my unnatural
birth stories

~ Alicia Jo Rabins ~

HERE ARE THE BIRTHS I didn't experience: The water birth. The home birth. The natural hospital birth. The triumphant release. The birth where I hold my wet amniotic baby to my chest and weep. The birth where I roar, poop, moan the baby out. The birth which leaves me knowing for the rest of my life that I'm strong and capable, that I can trust my animal body.

The problem with "at least the baby is healthy" is that, of course, it's correct. And yet, if there can be a "good" death, which I have seen and know to be true, then there can also be, not exactly a "bad" birth, that doesn't feel right, but at least a *worse* one. Even when the baby is, thank heavens, healthy. The problem is unclear thinking: We conflate the outcome with the process of the transition itself, whether it be the grief of losing someone or the joy of gaining a baby. When we touch the boundary between life and death, that quivering sphincter—wet and human on one side, black and empty on the other—we are electric. How we make that passage matters. How we open to make that passage for another being matters, too.

Here are the births I experienced: The anesthetic full-body shudder. The cold overhead lights. The freezing room. The strangers in blue masks. My strapped-down arms.

Two very different caesareans.

The first time was in Brooklyn, New York, a famously difficult place for natural birth. I hoped to deliver in the city's only free-standing birthing center, but at two weeks post-date I "timed out" and was sent to the hospital for an induction. That's late. The baby hadn't dropped, and it was right to be cautious. But on the other hand, I was born late, so was my husband; daily fetal non-stress tests and ultrasounds showed plenty of fluid and no distress. Still, the midwives said state law required me to go in. If I didn't, they warned, they would make it clear they were assisting against their will. So against *my* will I went to the hospital for a Cervidil induction. For twenty-four hours, nurses came in and out saying, "I'm going to up the dose," "I'm going to lower the dose," "Why did they lower the dose, it was about to happen?" After twenty-four hours of no food or drink and unproductive contractions, I gave in. The OB swept in, brusque, pissed off that I hadn't assented earlier. I was cut open just in case. My daughter was perfectly healthy. I was blessed, and also, wounded.

The day after I first gave birth, in New York, a birthing center midwife came to visit me in my shared hospital room the size of a closet. I was still in shock, sitting on towels soaked through with my blood, staring at the ugly gash across my belly. "This is the fun part," the midwife said, eying me and my newborn. "My kids are ten and twelve." There was something cynical and defeated in her tone, something beneath the surface that I couldn't identify. All I knew in that moment was that she had let me down. Later, I found out that she and another midwife at the birthing center had lost a baby a couple of months before I was due. The risk is real, too. The crossing can be perilous. It is important to acknowledge this.

Important to be grateful for the knife and the anesthesia when they can save your baby's life, or your own.

By the time I was pregnant with my second, we had moved to Portland, Oregon, where I was born at home thirty-seven years earlier. I signed up with a wonderful homebirth midwife and a naturopathic doctor who knew the OB who had delivered me. We prepared my cervix with herbs and acupuncture, and this time, a week after my due date, I slowly went into labor. That morning is one of the most cherished of my life. I walked around the neighborhood, knowing my son would be here soon. The next two days are a blur of pain and gratitude. I woke throughout the night with contractions, my water broke under our apple tree, I moaned in the birthing tub. After two days and only four centimeters dilated, my midwife suggested we go to the hospital for an epidural, so I wouldn't be exhausted during pushing.

And though I dilated fully (thank you, cervix!), the baby's heart rate began to decelerate dangerously during contractions. The words began to accumulate: fetal distress, heartbeat dropping, not recovering. I heard these words around the hospital bed and saw arrows pointing me back to the operating table. Simultaneously, amazingly, the epidural began to fail, and I was soon in thrall to one unrelenting massive contraction. The only relief was to push, but I was not allowed to push, because it made my son's heart rate go lower and lower. I felt my midwife's hand on my back: "She feels hot." More words through the pain: fever, danger, infection.

Naked on my hands and knees on the hospital bed, hugely pregnant, surrounded by strangers, my son's head halfway down the birth canal, wires and needles connecting my arms to the machines, three days into labor, overtaken by a pain so overwhelming I could only beg for relief. That was when they called the C-section. When he came out, my baby was blue, his Apgar's were three and ten, his cord gases were at the bottom of safe levels.

I was wheeled back into the room, and as I wept, the midwife said, "Yes, there will be tears." I tried to explain I was not crying because of the C-section. At that moment, I didn't care about the C-section. I was crying because my son was so exquisitely beautiful.

Afterward the midwife said I might have been able to push him out safely or use the vacuum extractor, but only if he came straight out, no upturned chin, no stuck shoulder. And babies do get stuck.

"He was all tangled up like a Christmas ornament," the OB said while the intern sewed me back up. I lay with my arms straight out, a horizontal Jesus, shivering from the anesthesia.

In the moment they called the C-section, I didn't care. In fact, I was glad. I just needed the pain to end—an animal need I couldn't control. I couldn't sign the release paper; I just waved my pen toward it. Writing was something humans did, and I was not human in that moment.

"My one regret," my midwife said later, "is that the epidural failed. I know you think you gave in out of pain." And then I did burst into tears for the birth I'd hoped for. "I wouldn't have let you do that," she said. "You knew to trust me. I was telling you it was no longer safe to labor."

And it's true. Pain or not, I would make the same choice again for my son. I would sign that paper. I wouldn't gamble his health for my birth experience.

Two caesareans, and yet I still believe in natural birth.

Why didn't my daughter descend? Was she in danger, or just waiting until the right moment? Why was my son wrapped in his cord? Could I have pushed him out or would he have gotten stuck, his brain damaged, worse? Why was I blessed with easy pregnancies? Why was I challenged with difficult deliveries? Did modern medicine save my babies or damage me? No one will ever know. Time has closed over itself. My birth stories have been written.

My mother gave birth to me at home. When I got pregnant, she gave me a copy of *Immaculate Deception II*, a pro-homebirth book. But her labor was long, too, and I required a vacuum extraction. We both think she likely would have had a C-section if my birth happened today.

Something was taken from me, but no one will ever know whether that prevented a much larger loss, a terrible loss. How strange when joy and trauma are wrapped up in each other. Is this motherhood? My midwife said, "A necessary caesarean is an act of love on the part of a mother. You shouldn't feel like a failure, you should feel like an Amazon." I imagined that cross-stitched on a sampler.

I'm grateful that I got to labor the second time. Those sweet, terrible, all-encompassing pains that made me sing in the birthing tub were so different from the pain of the knife that made me the mother I am, twice.

"I'm excited for your birth," each midwife said to me at seven months.

I will always wonder if my story could have been different. I still believe in natural birth. I believe it is possible for other women. I believe it was likely possible for me. But I also believe I learned more from having a C-section than I would have from a natural birth. There is a fierce lioness power in holding your newborn baby above your surgical wound.

I am less preachy, more sensitive to the tone of the conversation. I know that a woman can do everything Ina May recommends, everything the homebirth activists recommend—twice—and each time the birth can run away from her. I know *that* woman needs a book, too. The C-section mother is a powerful mother. Whatever power a C-section mother loses by not pushing her baby out she gains through healing herself. I know this to be true. I have experienced it.

They say women with dementia remember their birth stories; I am not surprised. I might always think of that knife, that suction, those stitches, with a twinge of sadness. And yet my wise midwife is right. Love for my children opened my belly. Love for my children drew this horizontal line between my hips. Love for my children gave me these unnatural birth stories.

I want to hear yours.

on becoming a mother, years after delivering a baby

Jacinda Townsend

I.

My second baby came to me before my firstborn did. She came to me in a dream while I was pregnant—a bald, shiny-headed baby who spoke, politely, in complete sentences. My then-husband is Italian, and I am Black; I remember being surprised, when I woke, at the pale color of the dream baby's skin, her blond eyebrows. But those are the whys and wherefores of genetics, I thought. This baby has come to me in a dream, so she must be mine.

And then my firstborn was actually delivered, with skin already deeply olive and a copious amount of raven-black hair. Not, of course, speaking full sentences. Not nearly as carefree in spirit as the breezy baby of my dream; this baby seemed already to be serious and brooding, perhaps predicting the next mid-year election results or calculating the consumer price index.

But let's back up. I didn't know my firstborn, not for two hours, because I was drugged to the high heavens. After twenty-seven hours of labor, I'd been slit open like a hog. So, while first her father, and then a succession of medical personnel held this beautiful baby who had been curled up inside me, sharing my life for nine months, I bled into bandages. Vomited up painkillers. When they finally brought my baby to me, I couldn't hold her because I was lying on a gurney, and unable to move. A nurse put her on my chest, and I hummed the only song I could muster into my consciousness: the theme song to *Winnie the Pooh*.

II.

The first time I gave birth, I did not actually feel that I had become a mother. For a long time, the first few years of my firstborn's life, I kept reminding myself that it was me. I was the only one changing diapers, nursing, teaching my baby how to read and how to speak in French. I was the *responsible* one here, but I had to tell myself over and over.

Perhaps it's because before mothering, before pregnancy, before even twinkles appeared in either my, or my then-husband's eyes, I was handed down a cosmology of mothering that did not include one's body failing to do its natural job. In 1999, I spent a weekend at The Farm, in Summertown, Tennessee. The Farm is one of the longest standing intentional communities in the world. In 1971, a caravan of brightly painted school buses and Volkswagen vans left San Francisco and crossed the country to settle on that land. When I visited in 1999, some of these original buses were still there, resting amidst the pristine pines and grasses of western Tennessee. There also is the legacy of Ina May Gaskin, a mother of modern midwifery. "Birth is a holy sacrament that belongs to the family," reads a page on The Farm's website. "Birth is a natural process best performed at home surrounded by family and supportive midwives." Ina May Gaskin's daughter-in-law said to me, as she helped her own daughter grab onto both her hands, lodge her feet on her mother's chair, and turn a flip, "By not letting women push their own children into the world, we're depriving them of their power."

It wasn't a new idea to me. My mother had told me that she never felt as powerful as when she gave birth. My mother is a force, and was always a fierce advocate for me and my sister. She always offered this—that much of her mama bear instinct, her courage to divorce my father, her will to take on a racist system that was stacked against her and her mothering, time and time again, originated in the moment of my birth. "You'll see," she told me when I was a child. "After you go through all that pain and pushing, you turn into something else altogether."

For me there had been no pushing. None. My cervix had dilated to only eight centimeters before stalling there for almost half a day, as if telling me I just wasn't ready for all this. And for many years after giving birth, my parental psyche was just as timid.

I took advice even when I knew it was wrong, because I thought surely everyone else knew better. "You should start her with jarred fruit," her daycare teacher told me adamantly, when I sent her to school with Gerber's organic spinach. I brought jars of peaches, even though I'd read widely that babies should be started on vegetables to lessen their risk for childhood obesity. I let teachers—and even other parents—talk me into anything. I was pretending to be my daughter's mother, waiting for her real mother to show up and take over. I felt that I'd failed her in the most important moment possible—that penultimate moment of her entrance into the world, and that I was thereby ineligible for success in the moments that followed.

III.

Before my first child was born, I found a doula. Attended natural childbirth classes. Read book after book and website after website on the birth process. Signed all the forms saying I didn't want an epidural. I didn't want my child to be exposed to the chemicals. Didn't want her to be weighed down with drugged grogginess in her first moments in this life. I wanted to feel and be present for each moment of birth. I wanted to meet my daughter immediately. I wanted to hold her. I wanted to breastfeed her. Smell her. Sing to her. I wanted to say, "Hello, baby. Welcome to the world."

Here's what I didn't know. Though C-sections are called for, naturally, in about ten percent of pregnancies, in this country, they are given to a third of women. The politics surrounding the birthing industry have been written about at length; I will visit with them here only briefly, to say that when I called the hospital where I was to give birth to find out what their epidural rate was, I was stunned to learn it was well over 90 percent. Early on in my twenty-seven hours of labor, when things were going well, I asked if I could have my ECG monitor removed so that I could walk freely and help my labor along. "No," said the rather unfriendly nurse on duty. And, to my doula, she said, "Make sure that woman gets an epidural." My doula nodded. My heart sank. Still, I resisted an epidural for the first day or so of labor. It was only when my cervix dilated from four to eight centimeters over the course of a couple of hours, and the doctors in attendance said I would be ready to push in short order, that I agreed to the epidural that had been dangled in front of me like candy for the twenty hours just passed. I was worn out by then, almost semi-conscious. My doula and my then-husband had listened to me moan in pain. They'd watched me sob and vomit bile. After twenty-five hours of this, they were both perfectly fine with my having an epidural.

And what did this magical epidural do? It stopped my labor. Completely. That epidural became the epidural I'd need in order to undergo an emergency C-section. My daughter was removed from my body not long thereafter. I didn't get to see her for hours. When I did, she was placed on my chest, and even that was painful to bear, so close to where I'd been sliced open. I couldn't hold her, so it was a small blessing, I thought, that she was asleep, and I was completely unable to move. She would never consciously register that, at first, her own mother hadn't been able to hold her. We both just lay there, while I hummed. I couldn't sing. It would have hurt too badly.

Five years later, I found myself pregnant with my second daughter and in the same kind of rural, nonprogressive community where I'd given birth to my first. The last midwife with hospital privileges had just had hers revoked after a dispute with a doctor over her advocacy during a birth. Only one practice in town did VBACs. When I interviewed her, the obstetrician I chose from that practice seemed genuinely supportive. I never thought to ask her how many VBACs she'd actually done in recent years.

As the weeks wore on, and I approached my thirty-eighth and then my thirty-ninth weeks of pregnancy, my obstetrician's support began to erode. "She's breech," she said, of my second born. My other daughter. She scheduled me for a C-section date. "It has to be on a Thursday," she told me. "I only do these on Thursdays."

Meanwhile, this wonderful body of mine began to remember what it had done the first time. It got into place earlier, doing things fast and furiously. I began having contractions. Still, I avoided the hospital and I avoided my obstetrician, because I knew a slow laborer seeking a VBAC didn't belong anywhere near a hospital. My contractions became more intensely painful and frequent that Wednesday. I knew that my regular obstetrician didn't do rounds on Wednesdays, and I knew by then—because I had seen the other doctors in the practice—that they were more supportive of my VBAC plans. "I'll wait for that baby," one of them said. "I'm not sure Schneider will." Finally, when my contractions were only three minutes apart, I went to the hospital. But as my mother wheeled me onto the elevator and up to the maternity ward, the first thing the on-duty nurse said was, "Oh. You're scheduled for a C-section?"

"No," I told her. "I'm going to give birth."

My obstetrician wasn't on rounds Wednesday, but she was there. Dressed to the nines under her white coat at six o'clock in the morning, but there. After examining me and determining my cervix hadn't dilated, she kept me, on the grounds that my feet were swollen. My feet had been swollen for five months—I had made her aware—but she claimed she had, then, to do a twenty-four-hour protein test for preeclampsia. When that test came back negative, my obstetrician said she had to keep me another twenty-four hours because my blood pressure was elevated.

"Of course it is," I told her. "You're trying to slice me open like a hog."

Nonetheless, at the end of that twenty-four hours, I had managed to watch enough mindless television and drink enough water to lower my blood pressure—I had beautiful numbers. I had also lost my mucous plug, and during the course of a stress test, my daughter had actually tried to take a breath, revealing that she was in no fetal distress whatsoever. We were nowhere near the two weeks after my due date, and my body was working beautifully. My daughter was doing beautifully. Things were happening.

My obstetrician had an ECG on me during those forty-eight interminable hours, and my daughter's heartrate had been miraculously steady. Shortly before I was to be dismissed from the hospital, however, my OB brought in a chart showing that it had done one deceleration. One. One. "You keep throwing things at me," she said, though it was clear that she was the one throwing things at me. When told that I wasn't going to be on the C-section schedule that day, the anesthesiologist, an old man whose nose was crisscrossed with the telltale veins of alcoholism, came to try to talk me into having it. When I said no again, he sat there, in the visitors' chair at the foot of my bed, crossed his arms, and simply stared at me. Refusing him momentarily strengthened my resolve. But when he left, and I was faced with more mindless television and soulless hospital food, practicality crept into my brain. I'd already spent two days in the hospital and away from my older daughter, who was in her first week of kindergarten. I hadn't even had a chance to speak to her teacher. I can't explain it now, all these years later, but when I thought about it then, I lost all resolve.

I remember being so angry during the surgery. I was hostile to my obstetrician when she asked questions, hostile to that anesthesiologist who'd come to my hospital room to intimidate me. Even as my precious, beloved daughter was being surgically removed from my body, I felt an overpowering aura of hostility. I felt love only at the moment I heard my daughter cry for the first time. I felt a tear running down my cheek, and realized that, mid-surgery, I couldn't wipe it myself.

IV.

We fetishize the birth experience, as though those few moments will determine everything that comes thereafter. We take classes in which birthing is quantified and the moment of becoming a mother predicted. At three centimeters this, and at full dilation that, and at an hour after birth this. The fetishizing makes us do a series of if-then causation chains in our heads. "If I don't deliver this baby naturally, then I won't be able to deliver this baby vaginally. If I don't deliver this baby vaginally, then I won't be able to breastfeed. If I'm not able to breastfeed, I won't be able to bond. If I'm not able to bond with my baby, he or she will be doing heroin at age twenty." But truly, birth—or in the case of me and

my daughters, surgery—had nothing to do with motherhood.
There's absolutely no good-parenting flow chart that relates back
to the exact moment of birth.

I felt inadequate for years after giving birth the first time. What
began to change things were small moments of advocacy, tiny
bursts of mama bear. I removed my firstborn from one preschool
and then another when I felt things weren't going well. I con-
fronted children who weren't playing nicely with her on the playground, children whose parents were sitting nearby, allowing their
own sons and daughters to behave badly. I pursued, doggedly, a
diagnosis of gluten intolerance when I'd suspected it but no doctor
would believe me.

Perhaps one of the most pivotal moments was my decision to
leave my husband, her father, after a weekend of his screaming at
me. My firstborn was then four years old, and she'd been listening
to the screaming and watching the occasional property destruction
for years. That particular weekend, as my then-husband screamed
and slammed doors and threatened me, she sat on the stairs and
listened. I remember looking at her sad little face. "I'm going to
take this baby," I told him, "and just get in the car and drive."

"Thank you," my daughter told me, quietly. It was so simple,
yet so powerful. My four-year-old was expressing relief that I
would remove her from this situation, and so removing her was
what I would do, no matter how physically afraid I was, no matter
how unprepared. I would scrape together my savings and hire a
lawyer. I would put up with three years of vicious legal wrangling
with my ex-husband. I would do what I would do to protect my
daughter's psyche.

Finally, in the middle of those long nasty three years of ups and
downs, I had my second child, the carefree, bald daughter I'd
dreamed about during my first pregnancy. Time was tight and I
was still divorcing. I had started a new job and didn't have one

moment in a day to sit and think about my parenting. And, without even thinking about it, I accepted that somewhere, somehow along the way, I had become, quite solidly, the mother of two girls.

My second daughter was, in fact, that baby of my first pregnancy's dream. She was born so blond that she looked bald, and would look that way long after she began speaking. She was also the laid-back, younger sibling I hadn't birthed the first time. I'll never know whether it's just her basic inner constitution or whether she, unlike my firstborn, benefited from the fact that by the time I had her I realized that motherhood has nothing to do with birth.

It hits me sometimes, when I'm advocating for my children through bad school situations, or watching them happily eat whatever green vegetable I've served up and ask for seconds, that such moments of normalcy did not come easily to me. I'm reminded, at such moments, of all the years when every single act of my parenting was tinged with the feeling of having failed my daughter from moment one of her life. I used to wonder, back then: As long as you still carry the memory of living through an event, will you really ever get past having lived it?

Now, I know that you will and you won't. You'll remember having lived it, but your stronger memories will be of having overcome it.

V.

It's a warm spring day, and my firstborn—my eleven-year-old—is, somehow, impossibly, as tall as I am. She's just tested into the gifted program in the California city we're moving to and received praise from her cello teacher. We're on our way to pick up her six-year-old sister, who is already playing piano like a pro, who just finished acting in her first play, and who is as funny as any comedian.

And it's on days like these, days when I know that my children are happy and healthy and I've completely forgotten how they came into this world, that I know: We can fetishize birth all we want, but birth is one moment in a lifetime of parenting, and might even be the least of all the moments. Becoming a mother is not in the moment of birth: it's in the moments of love.

pulled into brightness

∽ *Amanda Fields* ◠

AT MY POSTNATAL CHECKUP, Cassandra, the midwife, plunged her fingertips into my stomach, which was pliable as a bag of wool: "Flex."

"I am."

"Looks like you have some work to do."

One could say that. The six weeks I had been recovering from a caesarean had been strenuous; a loose stomach was the least of my concerns. Still, the midwife's fingers arched into my belly, suggesting I was not quite in reach of an arbitrary line in the medical sand. When I told her my uterus had been jerking and jumping since birth, that it felt as if there were still a baby in there, kicking, that it startled me awake at night, even six weeks later, she shrugged.

Cassandra was one of nine midwives who might have been on call when I went into labor. I ended up seeing six of them during my hospital stay. The birthing center boasted an eight percent caesarean rate. I had planned to deliver there, in one of five rooms, with tubs, meant to replicate a home. Toward the end of my pregnancy, I had the gall to worry that I would end up in the floral room with the pink comforter, or that I would fail in my quest for a natural birth and ask for the light pain medication the midwives could offer, or that I would be stuck with Gigi, the one who always seemed fifty percent distracted by things other than the pregnant person before her.

My rosy concerns about labor and delivery deflated on the day I went over forty weeks. My daughter was low and ready, her head turned to the side and nuzzling in the birth canal, pleased as punch. A jellyfish pulsating in liquid, caught in sea fronds, where she stayed.

After a few days of induction, ripening, cervical checking, zero dilation, and many midwives starting and leaving their hospital shifts, it was Cassandra hovering over me as I experienced a cold, strapped caesarean and my daughter was pulled out. As I felt the dull pulls and tugs from behind the curtain, I turned a wedding ring over and over on a hand that squeezed mine. It anchored me, knowing my husband James was there, my eyes closed as I shook from the medication, and fear. I squeezed back and turned the ring. When I opened my eyes, I discovered Cassandra, her long slender fingers nothing like James's. Even now, though I know he was there, and I remember his worried face framed by a blue surgical cap, I can't position him in my memory. He says he was beside me. I know I saw him, but he floats. And soon, in this memory, he floats away from the OR with our baby.

In the birthing center, after checking my abdomen, Cassandra looked at my scar, which was ropey, thick, red, and ridged. "Start massaging it every day. Pick it up and roll it between your fingertips," she said. She claimed that this would not only help "break it up," but it would also prevent internal scar tissue from fusing my organs. I imagined the adhesions as an alien of muscle and blood and beating life. For weeks, I winced and practiced rolling the scar, an activity of simultaneous drudgery and pain that made me think of a dark coffee shop in Amsterdam, years before, where I had watched a tall man with dreadlocks roll the longest, thinnest joint in the world, with a deliberate precision befitting his state.

By two-and-a-half, my daughter knew the scar as the place she had emerged from. Five years later, it still aches and itches. It remains a searing reminder of failure, of a time when I fumbled with the question of grief, if I could call what I felt—after a full-term pregnancy, an unanticipated caesarean, and a healthy baby—grief.

Caesareans make up nearly 32 percent of all births in the United States. What was I grieving, given that one of my friends had birthed a premature baby years before that could fit in her husband's palm? For one, I faced the idea that my body wasn't strong or logical. I zombie-walked through the experience of surgical birth. Afterward, I felt I should have refused induction, or at least asked more probing questions about what was being done to me. Other caesarean moms went back to work in a few weeks, or strolled their babies in the sun a few days after their release, while every step I took was etched in pain. It made me feel excessively weak. Even so, the presence of other C-section stories has become a portion of enough.

Eventually, I visited a gynecologist about the scar. I had what seemed to be basic questions. Is the pulling and itching around the scar before my period normal? Why do other scars fade to a slight purple smear while mine sits on my skin like a damp cigarillo? What's going on with the internal scar, and how would I, or anyone, know?

Online, there were copious scar selfies in C-section forums. None looked like mine. On these sites, women would often discuss how fat they were, then post pictures of their flat stomachs. They addressed the group as "Ladies" and asked questions such as, "I've been dropping blood clots for two days, but my husband says I'm fine. What do you think I should do?" and everyone would

say, "Go to the doctor! Oh, my husband is so clueless, too. LOL!"
It was both 1950 and 2013.

When I revealed the scar, the gynecologist failed to hide a
cringe. "I've never seen anything like this. Keep putting Vitamin
E on it," she said, sending me on my way.

In the pale medical world, everyone and no one knows what
they are doing, or saying. We are puzzles only when standard
answers, sliding, gelling, and trying cannot suffice among the cur-
vatures and bites of our edges. If you've stopped bleeding six or
eight weeks out and have no sharp pains, you're fine, say the docs.
Meanwhile, in La Leche corners, the C-section scar is a succumb-
ing flag; the cloth diaper reigns; formula will leech itself like candle wax to your child's undeveloped digestive system.

After months of internet clicking, I caught a few lines in a forum
about keloid and hypertrophic C-section scars: ropey, red, raised.
My people.

"Oh, it'll be there for decades, maybe forever," said Doris, a
stranger I met on a plane that I was taking to Denver for a job I
wouldn't get. When you're a mother, you find mothers everywhere.
They will comfort you; they will judge you; you will tell them
intimate things.

~

While pregnant, I had done a lot of birth reading but eschewed
discussions about C-sections. I had bought into the narrative of
the C-section as either patriarchal imposition or emergency.
Besides, any thought of my organs splayed for viewing and rum-
maging, not to mention an epidural needle in the back, made me
feel faint. The "real" pain of vaginal birth had seemed a better
prospect, a pain generated by my body at some right time.

And, after the surgery and the return home, the baby on my
breast for hours, infinite squinting at my phone as I researched

the effects of C-sections, the increased risk for asthma, diabetes, on and on, and oh! how the baby did not get the vaginal secretions or fluids or hormones to keep her safe, and really, oh, how much better off babies born vaginally were going to be in life—after all that, a question sat like a stone in a riverbed: how different might my daughter be had she not been pulled into brightness, had she, instead, slid and stopped and started through the birth canal; or, even, had I remembered to insist that I do more than get a glimpse of her face, that I get to hold her, skin to skin, before she and James left me to get sewn up? Everyone remarks on the happiness of my child. Would she be morose if she had done the hard labor of moving through a ripened cervix rather than waiting, suspended, to be plucked?

I never helped her move. My cervix was a walnut shell, stinking and impenetrable. Several times after I had been induced, Gigi, the harried midwife, followed by Beth, the no-nonsense British midwife, snapped on gloves and tried to pull my cervix forward. At one point, Jean, the most directive of the midwives, informed me, with her hand plunged in, that the baby was bald (she wasn't). I remember these agonizing cervical checks the most: Gigi's hands, Beth's hands, Jean's hands tugging at a resistant, one-inch organ.

I had read *Ina May's Guide to Childbirth*, a stalwart promotion of natural birth. Had I fully worshipped at Ina May's altar, I would have placed myself impossibly far from medical intervention. I would have controlled external forces, allowing the ancient rituals of the female body to take hold.

This philosophy had been so convincing prior to the caesarean, but, with time, I began to sense the connections between this narrative of control and our nationalistic myths about choice, which extend to our policies and judgments. We live in a nation where, without any real blowback from the public, government representatives can make live statements about how those people who suffer from physical ailments have brought it on themselves and should not burden others' insurance costs. That thread of control—that we should be able to sustain slick bodies and defy the inevitability of breaking down—is a powerful root in birthing narratives that pit "natural" against "medical intervention."

For a long while, whenever prompted about my daughter's birth, I recounted the caesarean in an embarrassed apology. Everything I said was geared toward my body's failure: every organ that didn't function the way it should have, the brain that failed to resist, or even to think.

What I recall most from Ina May's book is a fascinating section about animals giving birth alone. When a birthing animal senses a predator, she can halt labor with a sphincter reflex until she feels safe. Flush with pregnancy, I conjured a furry shape in the woods, pain, a telling rustle in the distance, the shape clenching and ceasing, a pinched control in darkness. The sterile brightness of my caesarean brought those passages back. The baby had dropped. My body had been ready, but something startled my cervix. It had gone into hiding when poked. It wasn't time. I had never said it was time.

It was easy but maddening to think in such simple terms, which removed layers of context, the parade of midwives and nurses and doctors and surgeons, the blood and medication and needles. This thinking worshipped the binary of light and dark, the limited caverns of cold medicalization or womblike warmth. It made it easier to claim grief.

So, the questions rolled in. What would have happened had they given me a few more days, another week? I had been induced due to low amniotic fluid, something that I learned in my post-caesarean reading is a common rationale for induction when, wait, wouldn't the fluid be difficult to measure in a uterus filled with a baby? Wouldn't there be less fluid as the baby got bigger? I thought that digesting so much information was helping, that scraping the plate clean might give me answers. The readings inspired the guise of a disappointing truth, that, somewhere in the labyrinth of my birth story, I should have trusted my body to have a baby without intervention. I should have found a way to say no. The most difficult thing about this feeling is that its persistence can't be explained to anyone who says all that matters is that mother and baby are safe.

I dredged my memory for anything that felt like evidence of real labor. During one of the interminable cervical checks, a midwife broke my water. While an accident, the warm rushing felt as I had anticipated. And, in the morning before the caesarean, I had serious contractions. I worked hard, holding my stomach, leaning over the bed, bouncing on an exercise ball, trying to recall all the natural birthing moves I had learned. I was doing labor lunges beside the bed when a blood clot, quivering and thick, fell out of me. I slipped on it gleefully—things were moving. James looked hopeful, too. In the coming months, if I mentioned my disappointment that I'd never really labored, he would say that I had looked like I was in great pain. Yet, each time I felt certain something was happening, the nurse would check the readout and shake her head, and everything slowed. The contractions were a hoax; I was hooked up to a machine.

The second time Gigi came on shift, she said they would no longer be checking my cervix. "It's traumatized you." From a chair in the corner, my mother, discreetly clutching rosary beads and retaining no faith in midwifery, agreed. Gigi had a bowl haircut and a red, breathless face. In the time that I had been sitting in the hospital with my immovable cervix, she had delivered three babies. She revealed that the doctor on duty was recommending a caesarean, and I cried. She leaned in. If you were to eat, the doctor—that invisible man down the hall who has never bothered to look in on you—would have to delay surgery, and this would give you the night to get labor going. This wasn't something she had cleared with the doctor; she told me that my eating would be an innocent mistake, my responsibility. And I wondered, were we having a ladies' moment, the kind where we are supposed to be in cahoots against some man I had yet to meet? I don't know—I've never been a ladies' moment person—not with squealing gal pals or fellow feminists or any mix of genders steeped in group emotions.

That night, the doctor entered with Beth. He scolded me; if I hadn't eaten, we would have been doing a C-section at this moment. I thought of what Beth had said in the preceding days to try to inspire me: "It's Children's Day in Japan!" "It's Cinco de Mayo! What a wonderful day to have a baby!" The doctor, clearly aware that a midwife had sanctioned my meal, shook his head at Beth, who pursed her lips.

Another vaginal suppository, more Pitocin, an Ambien for sleep (Ambien! It was given to me as naturally as a sip of water, and I gave no thought to it, I who would normally avoid a single ibuprofen), and surgery in the morning if I couldn't convince my body to open up.

I was resting when a couple of the midwives and two surgeons emerged to tell me that a C-section was inevitable. I had met one of the surgeons before, during a second ultrasound I'd had since I was just on the other side of thirty-five, "advanced maternal age." When the baby had not moved enough for her, she punched my stomach hard with her fingers and said, "Come on!" Now that surgery was inevitable, she shook my hand with political fervor as I wept.

The surgery felt as if someone were slicing an apple atop my numb belly. There was a thump-thump when the baby kicked my

insides one last time. In the air, her brow was furrowed and critical. Then she was across the room, squalling. Then she was gone.
It didn't occur to me to hold her. Later, on Facebook, I would see
photos of happy C-section moms, their babies' heads nestled
somewhere around their sternums in front of a blue curtain, and I
would think, *Oh*. Over in the room where I had never labored, her
first photo was taken. In it, James is wearing an orange T-shirt and
embracing her swaddled body with ease, looking down on her
with lovely tired creases beside his eyes, hair adorably askew. I
didn't see her again until after they had sewn me up, after everyone else had watched her squall and get checked and had let her
squeeze their fingers with her pissed-off hands.

Over the next few days, lactation consultants trooped through
the recovery room with competing advice. My nipples bled and
scabbed, the baby flattening them as she worked out how best to
get milk. One of the consultants scolded the baby for "snoozing
and cruising." The baby and I would unhelpfully fall asleep every
time she tried to nurse, such a deep sleep that I would startle
awake, astonished that I couldn't perform the only job I needed
to do. James did everything else—walking her through the halls,
taking her to the nursery for check-ups, changing her diaper,
carrying her to me, dressing and swaddling her.

I felt I had somehow been tricked and could not rise to the
greatness of motherhood. I only performed functions that James
could not perform, and I was even rather bad at the breastfeeding.
Everyone else was taking care of the details. People checked my
vitals in the middle of the night; if I awoke, a nurse would whisper
gently to go back to sleep. Food came and went. People handed
me the baby and all the things I could not reach.

More bodily incapacities characterized these days in recovery.
When my catheter was removed, I cried at the prospect of walking
to and from the bathroom. I was told not to use my abdominal

muscles, so getting out of bed was a long journey. I would roll on my side and fall forward, then shuffle. There was a tight band over my abdomen, and whenever I had to take it off it felt as if my guts would spill out.

My body was a vat of liquid. Since my blood pressure was so low, an iron sucrose drip pulsed down my IV tube like maple syrup. I felt it in my veins, warm and slow. When a second dose was needed, one of the nurses decided to thrust it all at once into my IV. She blew the IV, and my heart rate went up. After an EKG and some time, everything was fine, but I had to pee, and no one would let me get up. The woman sent to check my vitals said I could pee in a bedpan. I told her I would overfill it. She laughed at me, so I enjoyed the sudden independence of pissing and not ceasing even as the bedpan overflowed and I found myself in pools of urine.

In "The Last Person You'd Expect to Die in Childbirth," *ProPublica* and NPR offer a disturbing study of the maternal death rate in the United States, which is the highest in the "developed" world, though sixty percent of these deaths could be avoided. I don't consider my stay in the hospital to be one of utter neglect or danger, but, before I read that story, I thought I had been at the end of my grudging about the caesarean. I had decided it was done. I had decided that the problem was really me; it was all about perspective. Yes, and no. My questions were reasonable. There were missteps that had little to do with accepting my fate.

~

On the day I was released from the hospital, I cried as a nurse removed my staples. "We're not going to kick you out," she said gently. But James was tossing our things together and taking them out to the car. His joy frightened me.

The next morning, at home, I doubled over. For eight days, I hadn't shit. I lay curled on the bathroom floor, my mother hovering as James held the screaming baby. She was hungry, of course, never sated. For the first time since the surgery, James told me I *had* to get up; I *had* to feed her. I watched his crumpling face. He had changed every diaper, listened to medical staff compliment him for doing things because he was a man (a nurse had claimed that most men "just sleep on the couch"), expressed jealousy that he could not himself produce life-sustaining milk. He had walked me to and from the bathroom, handed me pads and listened to plops of clotted blood. Every night he left the hospital for thirty minutes, bought a microwaveable sandwich and a can of beer from the gas station across the street, and imbibed in the parking lot before returning to change diapers, carry the baby, hold my hand as my nipples cracked, stroll her up and down the hallways so I could get a few more minutes of rest.

He was home now—ready to start our life with this child. I could see this in his eyes, the fatigue, the hope. He had cut his way to this moment; he had made mistakes; he bore a harrowing family history. And now he had a family, a child, a chance to make his own circumstances. His hope was born from a hard-won desire to be a faithful, and great, parent and partner. I'm not telling you this to make him sound like a hero. I'm telling you this because I'm still not sure if I could perform so well if the roles were reversed.

As much as I tried that morning, though, I couldn't help him. I couldn't straighten out my body. My intestines were a puzzle of stone. I bent on the bathroom floor and tried to perform an enema, without success. I crawled out and clambered on the bed with help, my body contorted. I nursed the angry baby—my nipples on fire, my insides stuck, my surgical wound threatening to split. I returned to the bathroom, and my own mother tried to give me the enema. Nothing was getting in there.

We went to the emergency room while my mother stayed with the baby. The car ride was interminable, every bump and pothole an occasion for pain. I begged James to slow down when we could not go much slower. We got stuck in admissions behind a person detailing her sinus infection, a person who could walk and talk with perfect ease. I heard myself saying things like, "Help, I need help," in a voice I had not known existed. The man who eventually wheeled me to a room as James filled out paperwork refused to help me get into the bed. He simply watched as I tried to roll upward, then he turned away and pulled a curtain.

Hours later, the ER doctor could barely get the tip of his finger in me. This, after I had heard birth and death in the rooms next to me, as I lay there writhing and twisted up, full of shit. Full of shit, yes, and trying to measure this pain against the elderly woman I had seen who had died a few rooms over, and the various and far worse things happening to people in those frigid rooms, and my husband, torn between staying with me and wanting to be with our newborn, my husband who finally lost his composure when he had to ask one of our friends for help.

"They should not have released you until you had a bowel movement," declared the doctor who admitted me at the end of the day. A room wasn't ready, but a car accident was on its way, so they wheeled my bed to the hallway and piled between my feet a breast pump and a gallon jug of the clear liquid that might help me shit. They left me in the busy thoroughfare, where James, who had gone home to see our baby, found me. I had to stay in the hospital until I could force out the shit. That night, what finally emerged was ancient, scorching, and foul as brimstone.

~

In those first weeks after returning home, I had a disturbing anxiety about breaking our newborn's neck. I worried about losing control of my hands, an accidental, abrupt motion, as she was sleeping at my breast. Even as I watched her chest rise, I would weep, thinking I had done it, like a chaotic god. On the sagging couch, wincing at the jolts in my abdomen, I was as powerful as the gods of the slice and pull that had split my uterus. Baby blues? Something more? I was grieving a labor and delivery that didn't turn out the way I wanted, but I don't know what that had to do with my daughter's neck. Perhaps it was a sick belief in imagining horror as a way of negating it. Perhaps it was a belief in the mysticism of false anticipation, the way other people believe in prayer. Maybe I've had baby blues all my life.

I had failed to do a thing I am engineered to do, something my mother did twice and her mother five times, without incident or intervention. I kept replaying those days in the hospital. I second-guessed the induction. I felt angry that I had complied, then I wondered how in hell one doesn't comply with medical advice presented as fact.

I relived the assessment of my "old" placenta that had encouraged induction and set me on the path to a caesarean. The placenta was an old lady; she had outlived her usefulness; she was taking up space in the nursing home of my uterus. A cavern of stalagmites; the baby a bat waiting for the moon to rise. I had waited too long to procreate, and, in spite of a healthy pregnancy, it seemed I suffered the consequences of being old in a decade of my life where I had never felt more alive or ready to have a child.

In the years since I gave birth to one of the most dynamic, weirdest, and coolest kids I have met, I've read and listened to many caesarean stories, though there are far more that need to be told. It helps. I know that those who preach natural birth are onto something—the caesarean rate is too high, and the medical field is far less willing and able to listen to what women need for all the reasons that reveal the failings of capitalism, those attempts to wring out all drops of dignity. At the same time, natural birth proponents too often fail to recognize problems with their tightly stitched narratives of independence and control. I will never experience an uncomplicated moment of acceptance about my caesarean, but I'm done feeling as if it would have been better to walk into the desert and squat until my body performed, as if it were entirely up to me or a circle of strong, chanting women to make everything work.

When I left the hospital with my daughter, it was May in the desert. Outside were saguaros, a coating of heat that would become a roar in June, the rush of Tucson traffic, and the stretch of mountains over the valley. The sky was a vibrant, cloudless blue.

I waited in a wheelchair at the curb for James to pull up in the car. The baby was beside me, on the ground in her car seat. Seeing and unseeing. Eyes bright and astonished since birth; eyes that still emanate a craze for life when she blazes out of bed each morning. As we sat at the curb, a bird in a sapling above us chirped, and my daughter searched for the sound. I watched this moment, this one of her many firsts, my eyes adjusting to the brightness. And it came to me that she had been with me through this, the whole time.

upside down

∽ *Mary Pan* ∾

ALL THOSE YEARS DELIVERING BABIES, a trained physician's hands at the ready, guiding the crowning head, gentle traction on the afterbirth's cord, sewing up the torn vaginal tissue; reapproximation, each stitch restoring the mucosa to its previous unshorn shape. When I was the one delivering the baby, I had control.

Then came my turn: swelling belly, persistent vomiting, ballooning breasts, healthy baby. On each visit, according to all the tests, everything was textbook. But then, almost to term, my baby turned upside down. Breech, they call it. Bottom first tucked in my pelvis. This wasn't how it was supposed to happen.

I knew right away what this meant: a caesarean section, an incision, a scar. As a physician who had delivered dozens of babies myself, I was well versed in the risks associated with trying to deliver a breech baby in the traditional way. Babies have the best chance for a safe exit from the womb if they are head down. Transverse or bottom-down positioning increases the risk to both mom and baby during delivery. My training informed this choice and fueled my intentions to advocate for a different outcome.

In residency training, our experienced Labor and Delivery nurses would hand us newly minted doctors the patient's birth

plan after she was admitted in labor. This plan, which summa-
rizes the patient's desires for their delivery, is laid out weeks in
advance, before painful contractions ensue. The mother-to-be
outlines a play-by-play of her preferences: who she wants in the
delivery room, whether or not she desires an epidural or other
pain medication, if she would like to use a whirlpool tub or a yoga
ball to help ease the pain, if she would like music playing in the
room; all the salient details. During my training I learned the
macabre adage that those who produced the lengthiest birth plan
were the least likely to have a delivery go exactly how they envi-
sioned. It was an ungracious attitude toward anxious parents-to-be,
but the experienced obstetric providers knew: The less you expect,
and the less you count on when it comes to how your baby will
come into this world, the better. Babies, even before they come
out, are unpredictable.

As a physician, I knew that I shouldn't expect every detail to
play out exactly as I wanted. And yet my role had altered. In
pregnancy, I was no longer on the providing end of medical care.
I was the patient. I had never anticipated a primary C-section
and I didn't want it. My own mother had three quick vaginal
births, ushering my two brothers and me into this world in record
time. It never occurred to me that I might have a complication,
an aberrancy that would lead to an alternate birthing path. I
became irrational, a physician who put aside all she knew in scientific fact in favor of anecdotes, hearsay, lore.

I tried to get her to turn. I was desperate. I attempted everything
the internet told me might work. Frozen peas at the top of my
belly, awkwardly pregnant handstands in the lap swim lane at
the pool, playing music near my pelvis to lure the baby's attentive
ear to the preferred nether regions. As a physician, I had been
trained to adhere to evidence-based medicine: carefully researched
treatment plans based on scientific fact, not the whims of

speculation. In my urgency to find a solution to my undesirable state, though, I resorted to that which I knew had no reason to actually work.

Of course, all I really wanted was a healthy outcome for my baby and for myself. I realized part of my drive was due to a subtle, sometimes even overt, cultural negativity toward women who have a caesarean. Even the language used: "Did you have a natural birth?" As if having a baby by C-section is unnatural. As if growing a human inside another human for nine months then caring for it the rest of its life isn't enough. The entryway has to be au naturel to reach the pinnacle of motherhood. As a driven Type A personality, I wanted only the highest achievement for me and my firstborn. In the world's eyes, that meant a vaginal birth.

My baby had other ideas; she was stubborn. My obstetrician tried to coax her to flip. He lubed up my belly like I was in a lewd wrestling match. The medication they gave me to relax my uterus made me edgy and vomitus. As a doctor, I had never administered this treatment to a woman, but I had read about it. The textbook explanation of possible side effects didn't align with the severity of my disequilibrium. There is so much in medicine we recommend and advise without ever having experienced the potential consequences ourselves. Adverse events, side effects, unusual reactions, pain, discomfort, fear: These all are experienced by the patient and lost in textbook translation to the medical provider. My pregnancy experience gave me empathy for patients, not only for situations involving maternity issues, but also for all of the other procedures and treatments I recommend or perform on those under my care. I gained a renewed understanding of patients' fear, their confusion, their need for someone to act as if illness occurs in a person, not a sterile vacuum.

With carefully directed massage, my obstetrician got my baby's head to move four inches to the left, his right. (Whose perspective counts here?) Whichever way, it wasn't enough. She wouldn't budge, her head bobbing back against my liver like an evasive apple in a barrel mid-autumn. I held out hope to the very end. But eventually they had to cut her out.

I walked calmly into Labor and Delivery that grey, winter morning; no contracting uterus, no water breaking. Just the pinch of the IV into my arm, the steady hum of the blood pressure cuff inflating every few minutes, ensuring I was ready for, and stable on, anesthesia. The sterile blue curtain, just inches from my face, blocked my view. All I felt was a vague tugging that heralded my baby's debut just beyond.

In all the excitement, they forgot to remove the dividing curtain, as they'd promised. Prior to the surgery I had asked about lowering the drape when they delivered the baby. My obstetrician, slightly hesitant, but conceding to me as a physician-colleague, had agreed. I'd assisted in many caesareans but wanted to witness something of this birth, my own. It was a last attempt to play some role in the birthing of my own child, strapped down and immobilized as I was.

Most women have expectations of their birthing experience: what it might be, how it might feel. I was no different. My disappointment at the disconnect between what I wanted from giving birth and my actual delivery was almost tangible, the realization of an expectation unmet.

I lay there numbly, blindly, listening to the rhythmic hum of the blood pressure cuff tighten and release around my upper arm. I held her, my daughter, as my lower innards lay open to the world: uterus sewn up, patted down, checked for any bleeding. They systematically put things back in place, the way it's supposed to be.

I stopped delivering babies after I had my own. This wasn't due to my experience of delivery in any way, but a practical necessity of new motherhood. My newborn daughter suffered complications her first day of life. She ended up being admitted to the Special Care Nursery for a week-long hospital stay. I didn't leave her side, puttering with her through the halls in my slippers and carefully curated nursing tanks bought months before. My daughter recovered fully from her relatively minor issues of jaundice and fever, but I couldn't help but wonder, *Did I put her at risk by having a C-section?* Maybe she wasn't ready; or my dates were somehow off; or she needed more time in the womb, in the safe confines of my uterus. Of course, I'll never know. And though my knowledge as a physician assured me that a planned C-section was the safest option for my child and for me, given the circumstances, I, as a patient, couldn't help but wonder.

Pregnancy and the aftermath are unpredictable, and I was as exhausted as any new parent. Over many years I cherished my role as an obstetric provider but, in the end, couldn't reconcile the erratic work hours with my new role as a mother. I still provide family care, counseling women on preconception, caring for newborns just hours old. Because of my experience with a primary C-section and the complications that my own child experienced right after delivery, I am better able to understand my patients' anxieties, their uncertainties about navigating a metamorphosis of body, of emotions, of roles.

Years later, my lower abdominal scar is still bumpy, more raised to the left. The scar is a little off; not quite straight, not quite centered. My symmetry is disrupted. This surgery, my first, branded me for life and changed me as a physician. In medical school we are taught anatomy and physiology and pharmacology, but we lose an aspect of our humanity, our vulnerability. We are confident, knowledgeable, factual. We communicate outwardly, but we often fail to really listen, to understand.

When we take a bath together, my daughter likes to run her finger over the rust-red scar. It's bumpy, tactile. Sometimes I wonder if the stitches are still lurking, just beneath, slowly making their way to the surface or migrating ever deeper, disappearing into my pelvis. "They had to pull me out of you, bottom first, upside down." She says it cheerfully, matter-of-factly; her bright eyes gleam, recalling a personal memory she could never actually remember herself.

"Yes, they did, Baby." I affirm her history, acknowledging the slanted scar. This was my initiation into parenthood and all it entails: the loss of control, constant questioning, and recurrent failures. My body, my careful plans, my life's moments, were no longer my own. Upside down and jumbled about, my daughter readied me for motherhood. She gifted me with a new perspective as a physician.

My parturition was an initiation into a better understanding of my patients. I learned the importance of being an empathetic observer, of acknowledging a difficult experience—the difference that can make a patient feel off-kilter and unsure. For those lessons in motherhood and in medicine I am grateful. Maybe that's the way it's just supposed to be.

wounds

∿ Robin Schoenthaler ∽

FOR THREE YEARS I carry my son Kenzie to new-mother groups on Friday nights or singing groups on Sunday afternoons, and often you ask me—you or your sister or your neighbor or your cousin—you ask of the baby papoosed to my chest or dandling on my knee, "Is he your first?" Each time it happens I look at you, at all of you, and blink and wonder: Do I tell this nice person, your nice cousin, your sister, your neighbor, do I tell you about Kenzie's darling dead brother, or do I take a deep breath and nod and move along?

Sometimes at these gatherings, one of you asks me about Kenzie's birth story and I mention his C-section and you tell me your story, or you or your sister or cousin do. Everyone has a story, an angry story, about an earlier C-section, or an unfeeling doctor, and a dream lost; a long story, full of blood and anger and guilt. "I had to have a C-section, too; I'm so bummed," you say, or, "I've felt like such a failure; I feel like I was robbed," or "I've gone through three OBs who won't let me VBAC this time," or, "I can't bear to look at my scar, it's like a wound on my womb."

And I have to stop and take another breath, maybe two, because I want to hold Kenzie up in the air in front of you all and tell you, "But this darling boy is here today because he was born via C-section." I want to stand straight up, tall and with hips jutting outward, toes turned out, gesture to my scar, tell you, "Look at me, look at us, look at this—this C-section scar saved my life. It's not a wound—it's a life door."

~

I want to say to you and your sister and your cousin and all the women who see a caesarean as a loss: A C-section for us meant life. His life. My life.

But first comes the life lost. The life destroyed and the soul shattered when the caesarean wasn't done on time, when, in a colossal misjudgment, an on-call obstetrician let me labor too long with my firstborn, my Ryan Peter, waiting to be born after a perfect pregnancy, but with his head jammed in my too-small pelvis. Ryan Peter was the baby who couldn't be vacuumed out and couldn't be forceps-ed out, and whose soft sweet skull bones could not protect his little brain, so that while still inside me, his brain began the process of bleeding him to death.

This is what happens when a caesarean happens late, when, for whatever reason, a doctor tiptoes around the "caesarean" word until there is no chance, so that after they finally open me up and spend ten minutes tugging and heaving and nearly tearing my pelvis apart; the baby they are finally, finally, finally able to wrench out is not breathing, not responding, barely has a heartbeat, and, even though a few minutes later he begins to whimper, and to breathe, and to wave his little hands about, they know, we all know, that he is ruined.

Within twenty-four hours, he's in a coma. At thirty-six hours, he's having seizures.

We baptize him at forty-eight hours as they slide a tube into his lungs. This lets him live long enough to become that rarity of all rarities: an infant organ donor.

This is what happens when you don't have a C-section as you should: my son Ryan Peter, my gorgeous boy, becomes doomed to a four-bed life. For a week, he sleeps in an incubator on a ventilator as his head grows three times its normal size. Then he rests on a gurney in a coroner's office for two days, awaiting the mandatory autopsy, which shows a brain filled with blood and clots and scabs from the trauma of his birth.

He will lie in a baggage claim container for a cross-country United Airlines flight while I sob uncontrollably above him in coach.

He will rest in a casket that looks like a blue bassinet and slides into the ground in the Mountain View Cemetery in Oakland, California, under an enormous oak tree that will eventually die in a drought.

⁓

This is what a birth and death by delayed caesarean looked like for me, a middle-class woman in middle America: a stunned survivor incapable of speech. For weeks, I sat unmoving and stupefied. I had done this all alone, a single mother by choice, proudly pregnant and glorious in labor, but now I was as alone as I've ever been.

But this is what birth looks like eighteen months later, when I give birth again via a miraculously easy C-section. My obstetrician Sharon—who will eventually see me through five succeeding pregnancy attempts and three miscarriages, each more soul-splintering than the last—suggests we schedule my second son's C-section for thirty-eight weeks, since we "don't want to take a single risk with this one." We sit with a calendar and count back

from my due date. I pick the earliest possible day—January 4—
forty weeks minus fourteen days. I know it is too near to Christmas, but all I care about is being done, being safe.

Nineteen years later, my son Kenzie complains every holiday—
it's too close to Christmas, all his presents are afterthoughts, he
gets no parties. I look back from the vantage point of the long,
ensuing years and think, *Why didn't I schedule it a week or ten days
later?* Grief makes you self-obsessed. You can't imagine a teen boy
morose. You can't imagine anybody as morose as you, ever.

~

Sharon tells me the caesarean will be slow and long. There is
probably a bit of scar tissue and the baby is big again, but things
will be orderly, accounted for, attended to, addressed. This is not
an emergency C-section after hours of pushing; this is an 11 AM
section, second case of the day, with a doubled-up staff, no stone
left unturned.

My parents arrive two days early, a long enough time to help set
up the crib I had refused to pull out of storage, short enough so we
have only a little while to wonder. We drive through a Boston winter landscape to my final ultrasound appointment.

"We know what we're getting into. We won't take any risks,"
Sharon intones again. Everywhere we go, we see disasters: cars
stuck in snow banks, people's slip-and-falls. We know they're not
omens. We are inside of a circle of catastrophe; its aim, on others,
at last. Not us. Not us.

Kenzie's caesarean is stately, majestic, simple. There are twenty
minutes of preparation. The chief of obstetrics is there, murmur-
ing and humming. My parents and two friends are there. The
nursing staff and two pediatricians pack the room; half of them
had been there with me for Ryan.

My eyes are wide open, but I'm resting deep inside the base of my skull. I am gazing at my brain stem, willing it to stop on command—stop the blood coursing through my veins and arteries, stop the exchange of gases, lower my blood pressure to imperceptible—and to do so the moment I say to, because although I am lying there quietly, I know, deeply and suddenly, that if my son doesn't live, then neither will I. Women are meant to die with their children in childbirth, and this time I am ready to go.

~

Sharon's frets turn into cooing as she lifts my son aloft, into the lights above us. A circle of white surrounds him like a halo and I come running out from the base of my brain and am all cheeks, eyes, lips, gazing at my son. They wipe him off and place him on my chest. He inhales and gurgles and turns to the sound of me, gasping.

Kenzie stares at me while people leave the room. He glances away only when Sharon calls, "I'm starting up the stitching." It's the same incision as Ryan's, but this one with lightweight sutures delicate as lace, interrupted only on the occasions when she has to ask the scrub nurse to dab away the tears in her eyes.

Three years later, I'm in the same delivery room with the same yellow paint and white-blue lights. I have shooed all witnesses away; my friends and family are in the hallways so I can concentrate on nothing but this birth. Sharon is the OB again, and she knows exactly how to cut and tug my last son out without a bit of hesitation or pain. This time she lifts him up in the air gleefully. My whole being reaches for him.

And then I am clutching him to my chest.

Sharon stands straight and tall and thrilled, and, while I watch her sewing me up, I come to realize that in a different century or in a different country or in a world without the Sharons, childbirth would have been my death. I would have died with either Ryan or Kenzie—I would have died like the women I saw in Africa when I worked there as a medical student. I would have pushed until I burst or bled out or simply weakened beyond breathing.

I lay there holding my darling Cooper, remembering those bleached and ashen women on the Serengeti. If it hadn't been for Ryan's caesarean, I would have worn the same label they did— "died in childbirth." I would have become a statistic instead of an ecstatic mother in a delivery room. *I would have labored with my children until I died.*

In medical vernacular, I have now been "gravid"—pregnant— six times, and delivered of child ("para") three. In obstetrical shorthand, I am G6P3; a phrase of breathtaking asymmetry. Six times now, my womb has been emptied of its contents—three times sliced at its narrowest dimension, and then thrice resewn with sutures of fish-gut and lace.

The room is bright, and Cooper shimmers in my arms while Sharon sews me up; this time it feels like fireflies fluttering around my hips. From a long-ago bereavement book, I remember a Rumi quote: "The wound is the place where light enters you."

I say it aloud and watch Cooper's eyes light up at the sound of my voice. I'm shudderingly grateful for the wounds that have saved and healed me, and poured life and light into the eyes of my sons.

birth geographic

∾ *Aimee Nezhukumatathil* ∾

1.

When you give birth, there is no map—no bud and burst of compass blooming in the corner of the page. How do you know where to visit?

2.

My mother had a Caesarean. I had a Caesarean. My son will not have a Caesarean. He will glance up at the lights in a dentist's office and think only:
Lights.

3.

Suppose you had a ball at birth. A literal ball—one you could hold in your arms, bigger than a beach ball. I brought my very own to the hospital. Mine was rubber, a good weight, blue. A whole planet beneath my legs. Nowhere in that world was it cloudy. In between contractions, I rocked and rocked on the Earth and it was good.

4.

[[In the Philippines]]

It is said that if a woman has a lot of blemishes on her face, the baby will be
     a girl.

It is said if the mother glows and radiates beauty, the baby will be
a boy.

It is said if a mother is craving sweets and other carbohydrates, the
baby will be a girl. It is said if a mother is craving oily or fried foods,
the baby will be
     a boy.

> *I only craved sleep, so I thought*
> *for sure I would give birth to a pillow.*

It is said the mother cannot eat anything slimy or she will miscarry.

It is said the mother should eat fish (especially bangus) to make her
child
     smart.

It is said the mother should not eat mango to avoid having a hairy
baby.

> *Oh, dear heart—*
> *I fear we may have a very smart and terrifically furry child.*

5.

[[In India]]

My father was the first of six children born at home, in the
kitchen, surrounded by tin bowls and cups, cinnamon, and coriander.
It was an easy birth. He was an easy child. This is all I know from my

grandmother. I once tried to ask him about it when I was first pregnant: You were born in the kitchen?

—Yes.

His cockatiel squawked in the next room. He brought it to his shoulder. It sat there while my father continued to read the newspaper.

And that is all I know.

6.

When a female bower bird arrives to inspect the male's nest, the male struts and sings. He hopes his carefully decorated entrance and "avenue" will entice her to stay. To this end he selects all manner of blue decorations to line his nest: pen caps, flower petals, berries, chips of shell, bits of foil. All blue. If the female leaves—he will simply wait, hope for her return, and pass time by constantly fine-tuning the placement of each knick-knack, each twig and snap of branch.

7.

I had   a birth plan—Xeroxed and stapled, slipped   into

     a manila folder   for easy distribution   among

          the nurses when I arrived at the hospital. I had a

doula   who

was supposed to "hold

the space" for me.   Everyone slept.   Even the doctors.

     Everyone slept   except my valiant husband

who stayed awake   for almost three days

and stayed   strong as a pepper plant.   He was starlight

and samosa and every good thing.   I could actually see

him   even though I had my glasses off. My three-page

single-spaced birth plan shrank   into one sentence—"Mother alive,

baby alive." And when my husband wasn't looking, I snipped it

to just two words:

8.

Baby alive.

9.

Oh where was the Knight of Knives to rescue this lady in the high
tower? Where was the sword, the halberd, the red banner?

It was my decision. Mine alone.

10.

No one suggested   I get it done. No one even whispered it,

or maybe they did—

but I never heard it. I would have fire-screamed them out

of my sight. After thirty-two hours of labor

and no drugs, my tiny body frame

simply gave out.   I pushed twice and leg-wobble.   More leg-wobble. I looked at my husband   and he nodded *Yes.*

    I was a table with no legs,

on a table with no legs, transferred   to another table and

bitten

in my back   like the bite of lemons

        in your first sweaty drink of the summer.
Delicious.

11.

My mother promised me her special dessert when I finished, so I
focused on that: alligator pears (avocados) mashed with milk and
sugar, a little dollop of ice cream.

12.

When I couldn't focus on sugar, my husband held my hand in front of
the blue curtain and when I felt the tug—I focused on his sweet face.
All the chrome and shine in the room could not match the brightness
of his smile. I was a fish, a happy fish. I finned up to meet his face. My
husband was all the bright lure I needed until I was caught. When I
was caught, I didn't put up a fight. I lay there and let them do their
beautiful job.

13.

Memorial Day weekend: everyone was supposed to be at the beach
for a picnic. They hauled me up for the double chord and catch. And
inside me:

        a boy who I promise you, smelled like the sea.

14.

Directions for Assembling a Bluebird Nestbox:

    a. Position one side approx. ¼ inch beneath the slot flush with
        the edge from the back and nail from the back.

    b. Nail the other side, taking care that both sides are even.

    c. Position the bottom centered on the nail holes and nail
        through each side. The top will be higher than the sides. This
        allows for ventilation.

    d. Slip the beveled edge of the roof into the slot and screw it
        down tightly using a #8 ¾-inch brass round head wood
        screw.

15.

Because I know talk like this frightens you, I will say this only once: If
I am ever lost or someone ever wonders if the cause of my death is by
my own hand—let it be known that I will never leave you on my own
accord. Never. If someone takes me, I will scratch and bite until I
gargle soil. My mouth will be an angry mouth if anyone rips me from
you. The center of my hands boiled with blossoms when we made a
family. I would never flee that garden. I swear to you here and now: If
I ever go missing, know that I am trying to come home.

16.

Oh, *Lord.*

Lord, my bottom lip is bruised from singing Your name.

But it is good, Lord.

We are good.

17.

All weekend long the dahlias spun themselves into creamy blossoms in the rain-slicked mulch. What flower should I call you? You arrived too late to be crocus, too early to curve into morning glory. Here in our tiny town in western New York, I was ready to give you anything—a dogwood branch, a solar system, complete with glittery meteors to track. A single orange. A dark and lucky sharktooth.

18.

Baby, we are *alive.*

PART TWO

At the Threshold

Caesareans save lives, but it hasn't always been that way. Though the surgery appears in ancient art and folklore from all over the world, it wasn't common until the twentieth century. By then, anesthesia had made it possible for surgeons to operate with greater precision. Aseptic suturing techniques allowed safe closure of the uterus, and antibiotics eased the risk of infection. Most importantly, birth began to move out of the home and into the hospital.

In 1970, the US caesarean rate was only 5 percent; by 1988, it had risen to 24.7 percent.[1] What explains the increase? Among a complex mix of medical and technological transformations, several stand out. Widespread use of the horizontal incision or "bikini" cut made it possible for most women to stay awake during delivery. Without a cut through major abdominal muscles, recovery was easier, too. Electronic fetal monitoring, common by the 1980s, allowed doctors to track a baby's vitals on screen during labor, but this technology changed the way we measure risk.[2] Birth scholars also connect the rise in caesareans to induction practices. One example is the use of Pitocin, which can intensify contractions and begin a series of interventions that eventually lead to surgery.[3]

In the US today, one in three babies are born by caesarean.[4] About half of these deliveries are repeat C-sections, scheduled ahead of time for a second or third child.[5] (Despite misconceptions, the rate for elective caesareans free from any medical factors remains low, at around 3 percent.)[6] And there are multiple medical reasons for first-time C-sections: Placenta previa, for example, in which the placenta covers the cervix so a baby can't move through the birth canal. Placental abruption. Cord prolapse. Breech baby.

CPD (baby too big). Preeclampsia. Placental accretion. Birth of multiples. Fetal distress. The most common reason: failure to progress in labor.[7]

The caesarean as lifesaver. The caesarean as birthing choice. The caesarean as surgery that reflects the history of modern medicine and significant changes in the way we give birth. Despite these changes, birth remains a threshold. Each time, it is crossed into an unknown. We give birth within intersecting webs of identity, culture, and meaning. What happens when we cross this threshold with C-section delivery? How does the experience ripple through our imaginations? The essays in this section speak to the real risks of childbirth and the intense transformation involved in becoming a parent. They explore the way that birth brings all of our relationships into heightened focus, how the process of bringing a baby into the world is rarely easy. Here, you will find writers imagining their way through connection and resilience as they recount their birthing stories.

the emperor's cut

∼ *Elizabeth Noll* ∼

BY THE BANKS of a great river, a woman lay bleeding, exhausted, and unseeing. The babies were lodged inside her—only one set of tiny legs emerged.

Beyond her were hills she could no longer see and horses she would never ride. Soft bedding turned red and sodden. Hands massaged her belly, wiped sweat, pounded leaves for medicine or poultice, perhaps beat drums. Tears came, and chanting, and whispering, and screaming.

They tried everything. But they couldn't untangle her twins. One breech, the other behind, entwined and trapped.

Her twins never got to breathe, and they took her with them.

She became a memory. Then she became just bones.

About 8,000 years later, they found her in a grave with the tiny bones of two fetuses still with her: one, half in and half out of her; the second, still inside. She died by the Angara River in Siberia.[1]

Her skeleton is one of the only examples of obstructed labor in the archaeological record. (As well as one of the few confirmed cases of twins.) It's very rare to find evidence of death by childbirth. Many women deliver before they die, and if they do die first, the fetus may be removed before burial. If the fetus dies inside the mother, its tiny, fragile bones might decay without leaving a trace. And without a fetus, there's nothing to indicate how the woman died.

There have been millions of women like her. But she was the one who landed in my living room, a traveler in a short paragraph on a glossy page. Archaeology is filled with pain from long ago and far away, but she was more than that. This Stone Age woman from the hills north of Lake Baikal—she was my flipside, my B-side, my what if, my abyss.

She was me if I'd been unlucky; if I'd lived in a different where or when; if I'd refused help or if there was no help to refuse.

A stuck baby stops the world.

That's one of the lessons I learned the day I had my C-section.

What I knew before
All through my pregnancy I said I wanted a natural birth. No drugs, no machines, minimal intervention.

I wanted to give my baby a pure beginning—the purest beginning possible, unpolluted by chemicals.

"Why? Why put yourself through that?" my husband demanded. "There's nothing wrong with taking something for the pain. If it was me, I'd be the first one in line."

We fought about it.

Our arguments were all about the epidural. We never once argued about a C-section. Chances that I'd need one seemed remote. My mom had five kids. Her mom had seven. My dad's mom had ten. None by caesarean. Green light!

I also argued passionately with one of my best friends. She tried to explain that there was a really good reason why epidurals were invented. That they were beneficial and not at all to be sneered at. In my arrogance, I shrugged off her good sense; in my ignorance, I couldn't really picture what kind of help someone else could give me.

At that point, I still believed that birth was ultimately a one-person job.

I thought if I controlled it all, nothing bad could happen. Nobody would have the chance to get in there and fuck things up. Because even though they say there's no harm in having an epidural, who really knows? Mistakes happen. What if there is an overdose? An allergic reaction? Some other tragic accident? No thank you.

Better safe than sorry. My plan was to just let that baby sail out and let Nature take care of things.

In my defense, there are a *lot* of stories out there about exactly that kind of birth. I even talked to women, in person, who said they *had* that kind of birth: incredible, awe-inspiring, full of joy. The kind where everything went right. The kind where, even though there was, technically, pain, (reluctantly admitted), it didn't really register as pain, because it was just the wonderful strength of the body doing what it was uniquely suited to do.

Growing up, I heard this about childbirth: "Oh, you forget all about the pain. When you see that little baby, you forget everything else." Always, the woman who said this was laughing. Maybe a bit nervously.

This turned out not to be true at all.

What I knew that day

Not only did I not forget about the Pain, it is the thing I remember about that day. Or rather, the Pain was so powerful it shorted out my senses, so there wasn't much to remember, except that.

It began on a moonlit night.

At about 1:30 AM, the cervical plug—a cork of old blood—came out. Nausea hit. The contractions got harder. My husband was still asleep. At childbirth class they'd said lots of women go to the hospital too early, and then they just have to go back home. I didn't want to be that woman.

But at about 3:00 AM, I woke him, because I didn't want to be alone anymore. He was upset I hadn't awakened him earlier.

He drove me to the hospital. The moon was nearly full and the blue-black air was cool on my skin. My baggy old gray Goodwill shirt with the sleeves cut out was practically the only thing that still fit. It was Friday, the first day of October.

I had trouble standing during intake. Soon I was in a bed, and the doula was talking to me about what I could do while I waited for things to get worse. She convinced me to take a warm bath. It didn't help, but it was something to do.

About 7:30 AM, the midwife showed up. The midwife I'd seen throughout my pregnancy; the midwife who was supposed to be my ace in the hole, my key to a woman-centered birth. She did a cursory exam.

"Doing great! You'll deliver by noon," she chirped.

I never saw her again.

My cervix dilated to about eight centimeters. And no more.

At one point, a few tears came to my eyes.

The doula noticed. "What is it?" she asked.

"I just want it to stop. I'm tired of the pain."

She looked at me in disbelief. I don't remember what she said. I don't think she said anything. But her expression was clear enough. This is only the beginning, her eyes told me; this is nothing compared to the pain that is to come; you have no business crying *now*.

And what her eyes said was all true.

After hours of contractions, they said I might be dehydrated.
They wanted to put in an IV. The doula reminded me that once
the IV was in, I wouldn't be able to move around.

But I didn't really want to move around, anyway. I
was exhausted.

They put the IV in. Then they wanted to attach the baby to a
fetal monitor. I'd been warned that the IV would be the start of
the medicalization of my baby's birth—the westernization of my
womb—and it was true: everything followed from that.

That's about when the Pain began.

My husband told me later that I was drenched in sweat. I was
naked and wasn't even aware of it. I was in agony for hours, but I
don't remember being in agony—I just know that I have almost
no memory of that time.

When the Pain was upon me, I could not see. There was no fog
and there was no dark. The lights didn't dim. There was simply
no seeing. I was too busy to see.

There was Pain, and Pain was all. The Pain replaced me.
It became me. The Pain took the place of my eyes and ears
and brain.

A pair of hands reached through. There were knuckles near my
eyes, to the right of the bed. I gripped the hands and they

gripped mine. How I knew I still had hands was that he held them. His skin was like medicine. It helped me breathe. Skin I knew. Hands I knew.

The Pain was in the room, but so were his hands.

Once—or maybe more than once—I looked up, very far up, and in the sky were his eyes. Worried.

Why is he worried? It was a question I couldn't answer. I couldn't think, and I couldn't speak.

Only later, when I trolled my memory for details, did I realize his hands were about the only thing I remembered from those hours.

I told him, "I don't remember much. I think there was someone screaming."

He looked at me. "That was you."

I think they gave me Pitocin, to see if it would make my contractions more useful—see if my cervix would dilate those last few centimeters.

After hours of that, they said I was exhausted and I should sleep. They gave me morphine.

I liked this idea. I wanted to sleep. But I couldn't. Something would not release me.

Someone said, "They gave her enough to put a horse to sleep."

It might have been my husband. He kept telling me I should
sleep. He got a little irritated that I wouldn't. He thought I was
being stubborn. He was exhausted, too.

But I couldn't.

There were murmurings, gentle threats. If I couldn't sleep,
somebody said, I might not have the energy to deliver, and there
might be a C-section.

But I couldn't. And after a few hours of that, something
did change.

Somebody said, "The baby is not recovering between
contractions." Somebody showed me jagged lines. They said,
"Look here, the baby is not getting enough oxygen."

That I remember—the piece of graph paper with peaks
and valleys, and the statement that he was in danger. That
reached me.

My husband told me later that doctors and nurses were massing
in the hallway, and eventually pulled him out of the room to talk
to him. They told him he had to convince me to agree to a
C-section. And they sent him back in.

My husband said to me, "We need to get him out of there. That's
the most important thing, that he's healthy. Right? We want him
to be OK. We want our baby to be safe. And he's not so safe right
now. He's not doing too well in there, so they have to go in and
get him out of there."

I whispered—of all things—"But you won't be disappointed
in me?"

That shocked me. Until I said it, I didn't know that thought was
inside me. I didn't know I cared that he might think I was weak.
Which was totally illogical. He had tried for months to convince
me to have an epidural; he clearly hadn't wanted me to endure
any of this.

"No." He shook his head. He was, perhaps, a tiny bit amused. He
told me I was brave and strong. He told me I'd done all I could
do. It was time.

So I agreed.

I don't remember my friend sobbing at my side when she realized
that, after all our late-night arguments, I was going to have to
have a C-section.

Into the wilderness came a man with a needle.

I had to sit up. Barely conscious, limp with pain and fatigue,
drenched in sweat, I had to sit up because the spine must be
vertical for the epidural needle to enter properly.

I understood this. The only way out of Pain was to sit up.

So I did it.

I didn't feel the needle going in.

Then I could see. Suddenly there were colors. I could see. I could
hear. I could talk.

The world was the world again.

I looked around for the miracle worker. The anesthesiologist was
standing behind me. I twisted all the way around, still sitting on
the bed.

"Thank you," I said, shaking his hand.

Before the birth, I'd read about epidurals. They sounded
horrible. Who wanted a giant needle jammed into her spine?
And the possibility of things going wrong—what if they gave me
too much, and it harmed me—or the baby? And the fact that it
didn't take all the pain away, but only 60 to 80 percent, made it
seem not worth it.

I hadn't read anywhere that an epidural can pluck you from
nothingness and give you back your speech and your sight and
make your brain work again. Nobody had written that about it.

Then I was in a big room. There was a lot of blue-green cloth.
My friend was next to me, taking pictures.

Then there was a pause. And a clump of doctors and nurses at
the far end of the room. I sensed they were done with me. They
must have eased the baby out. But there was no cry.

"Is the baby okay?" I asked. "Why isn't he crying?"

Nobody answered. I felt the beginnings of panic.

"What's wrong? Is the baby okay? Why isn't he crying?" Why wasn't anybody talking?

Later I found out they were giving him oxygen and rubbing his chest.

And then . . . a wail. A lovely, spidery, scratchy yowl. My friend said the doctor slumped, visibly relieved.

Sometime later I was in a small room, and that's when I got to hold him. He had on a little hat—blue and pink and white. He was all there, and he was out of me.

That's when they told me what happened. The cord had been wrapped around his neck twice, and as a consequence, it was too short. He would not have made it out of the birth canal.

What I knew later
I knew that a C-section saved my life and my baby's life.

I knew that pain can wreck a person, physically and mentally.

I knew that my failure of imagination had put me at risk.

I knew that the reason people help during childbirth is because the pain can disable the mother; because they can see things she can't; because they can do things she can't. It's nothing like the movies, where everyone else in the room is incidental and the woman huffs and puffs until the baby pops out.

I would not be sitting here, writing this, if we'd let Nature take
care of things. My son would not be asleep in the bedroom. We
would be just memories now. Memories and bones.

We think of the caesarean as a modern invention, but it's not. It's
been around longer than books. C-sections were performed in
China 3,000 years ago; in India 2,000 years ago; in Iran about
1,000 years ago. African tribes routinely performed C-sections in
the 1800s, and most probably long before that. Roman law
required that a baby be rescued from a dead mother's womb. So,
the first, and for a long time, only, use of a C-section in Western
civilization was to save a baby whose mother had died, either in
childbirth or from some untimely accident. It took centuries for
Western doctors to figure out how to do a C-section on a living
woman; even longer to figure out how to do it so that she
remained alive when it was over.[2]

In many Indo-European languages, the name for the operation
translates as "emperor's cut." (In German, for example:
Kaiserschnitt.) Oddly, though historical records show that Julius
Caesar himself—whose name the procedure carries—could not
have been born by C-section.[3]

Recently, C-section rates in many developed countries (China,
Brazil, the US, Australia, and much of Europe) have
skyrocketed. In some regions, C-sections are more common than
vaginal birth.[4] However, the increase in C-sections is only half of
the story. Each country's C-section rates are highest for the
richest part of the population and lowest for the poorest people.
In other words, women have unequal access to C-sections. Some
women have to fight to avoid the procedure, while others cannot
get it—including millions for whom the operation would be
life-saving.[5]

The World Health Organization did, at one point, declare that the optimal rate for C-sections was 15 percent. However, in 2015 they did a 180. Now their official statement reads:

"Every effort should be made to provide caesarean sections to women in need, rather than striving to achieve a specific rate."[6]

Of the estimated 18.6 million C-sections performed globally in 2014, about one-third are thought to have been medically unnecessary.[7]

Far more tragic are the estimated 3.18 million that were needed, but not performed.

~

When I think of a C-section, I think of light.

Because the next day, I got to go outside. Yellow-gold sun shimmered around the wheelchair as my husband pushed me along the sidewalk. The breeze kept yanking my hospital gown open over my thighs.

"You might want to, uh . . . " he said, gesturing at the flapping cloth.

I laughed. I held down the edge of the gown for a little while, but really, I could hardly be bothered. The air. The sun. The grass. The wind. All delicious.

My baby was asleep with the nurses and I was rolling along the banks of a great river.

a thin blue wall

~ *Jen Fitzgerald* ~

The blue was so calming, even in its intense contrast from the white and trans-lucent ice. I don't know what brought me to that place. There was a strangeness to imagining how it would all end, even then, in those final moments.

Between the ages of three and five, I have memories of being carried down the narrow flight of stairs from our apartment above a biker bar. My father would scoop me up and take me out of the house, away from my stepmother after a fight. She believed he was doing it to punish her. At the bottom of the steps, my father had cut a square hole in the wall to access the apartment's phone line wires. He would pull the phone lines apart in a well-worn spot where the wire had been stripped of its casing, and the frayed metal had been twisted around itself to reestablish connection. I don't know what the fights were about, just that they were a constant. In the beginning, he would ease the sheetrock back into place, but as time passed, he just left the wires exposed.

My stepmother later admitted that she knew about the phone lines and would reattach them after my father had left. It was a dance they did. He wanted to control access, and she let him believe he did.

That landing, too, was about access. It was the spot where my mother would stand many times, sobbing, arguing, denied entry, and me not being let out, moved as a pawn on a chessboard. I would see the door close on a figure descending the steps, never even knowing that she had come for me.

By the time I entered kindergarten, I believed love of that intensity to be dangerous. It left you open, vulnerable. It created an opportunity for you to act out of desperation. I would know better than to love like that.

A mother's love seemed to be the most dangerous because it was all pervasive and unconditional. Unconditional love was a seam showing through the coat, a thread that could be pulled to unravel the garment until you were naked. *If you show them how much you love the thing, they will take it away until you give them what they want—they will always be able to take it away.*

I believed I would be safe if I never got married and never, ever had children.

Blue is attention and ease—it is both natural and yet eye-grabbing when found anywhere in nature. How can something so natural also feel so foreign? Blue is the part of us that remembers we are more than a body, more than a vessel; we are the infinite contained therein.

⌒

I found out I was pregnant while escorting a friend and her infant daughter out of state. She was going to the site of a forthcoming writer's residency to prove to the board of directors that she could handle said residency with a baby in tow.

I knew the literary world to be a hostile environment to parents. I was also shown that *motherhood* wasn't something that belonged in poetry.

I found out I was pregnant less than twenty-four hours after my husband's uncle passed, due to an egregious surgical error—an event by which we now mark time.

I found out I was pregnant while living in an uninhabitable home undergoing a gut renovation.

I found out I was pregnant after a lifetime of pregnancy and motherhood being an unfathomable and frightening abstract.

All of this is easy to say—what I don't want you to know is, the night I found out I was pregnant, I laid in bed with my hands over my stomach, hoping that whatever was inside could feel the warmth. I promised that if it decided to stay, I would love it more than anyone had ever loved anything.

Fairly quickly, pregnancy "just started happening" to me. If I didn't take it day-to-day, careful not to dip below the surface, I would be wading in the muck of my childhood. I needed to go on instinct, rely on something primal to help me reinvent the way a baby is cared for, when, of course, I allowed myself to accept that I would soon be caring for a baby.

I could do the brick and mortar of it—I could get the furniture, clothing, bottles, diapers, and physical necessities. Those were distractions; emotion was akin to a flood. As I lost control over my body—hormones, stretching, creaking, leaking—it became harder to swallow the feelings of vulnerability. I was defenseless (even against a large gust of wind). How on earth was I supposed to protect the small creature inside of my body from the dangers seen and unseen?

Disassociating is a survival technique—once the body learns it, the body uses it, without permission, any time stressors are introduced. I cannot pinpoint the exact age at which my body learned to disassociate, but the muscle memory is vivid. There is a brief section of time between anger and rage. You can prepare and brace when you can pick up on that shift. I was at my most aware and most deadened in those spaces of realization, when I knew I was going to get hit or have objects thrown at me. I entered a state of being adjacent to my physical body, a space where I could witness what was happening but completely deny that it was happening to *me*.

There is one instance that resonates with me even now. Cornered, at the bottom of the steps, with no opening large enough on either side of my stepmother's body to see light, I learned and enacted the extinguishing of outer light just as she learned and enacted the extinguishing of an inner life. Not enough made it through for either of us to run toward if we'd ever get the nerve. A voice from within called, *go somewhere else*, and I listened. In this dissociative space, my physical reality severed. I tried to shield my body as the intensity of the present made me aware of a shared rage. Neither of us were good stewards of victimhood; we consumed, swallowed, and absorbed. Instead of seeing the outer-world as a reflection of the inner, we believed the outer-world was so chaotic because of some deficit, some inner lack. We were adrift; anger may be a reliable compass but rage capsizes. I don't know how long rage kept me trapped there; time loses its linear drag in an altered state.

When my therapist asked the "adult me" how often these incidents occurred, I had a difficult time pinpointing a number—the truly traumatic moments are accessible but there are so many I feel the large, steel door of memory shut over when I seek them out. Were the bad ones once a month? For eight years? Were the "not so bad ones" really not so bad?

As little as I understood the emotional well-being and upbringing of a child, I could go back into my own past and create a list of *never*. Never would I incite terror in my child. Never would I hit

her. Never would I make her feel unsafe. Never would I give her
reason to run and retreat mentally or physically. Never would I
allow her to live in violence. Never would she doubt her worth and
importance, never. This list represented survival guideposts. I
could navigate between them, careful never to get too close. Even
with these, I still didn't know how to love a child or how much of
that love to show the world.

If I swore to care for the child better than any child had ever
been cared for, but somehow keep my love for them secret, maybe
they couldn't be used against me. I could be aloof and yet effective,
right? I squeezed tighter and tighter as I swallowed more and
more. I shored up against the mounting pressure until my husband and I found out we were having a girl.

*The color blue brings peace; it pacifies and restores. It seeks out red and
warmth; it absorbs light and shifts from the darkness of navy to backlit, polar
ice. From the death hue of skin to the veins fueling the heart, it expresses life.
It radiates from within and from above.*

*When that blue surgical drape is lifted between you and your torso, your
mind and your body, and your past and future, you will find this divide permanent. A tectonic shift in your narrative pulses open doorways of the subconscious, possibilities of understanding. You will have to reemerge from this
division and find a new way to remain whole. There is no promise of peace,
but there is hope of healing.*

I was afraid to tell my father that I was pregnant. I have to turn to
stone when I talk to him, seize up so that no emotion can show
through. He was working on a towing trailer in my grandmother's
driveway when I pulled up. He'd created a world for himself
there, as he had with his own yards. His short frame was hunched
over the trailer hitch, and he straightened only slightly when he
saw me. I never knew where, in the kingdom of his inner world,

he was when I interrupted. This time I got a stoic greeting, other times he would feign affection or throw out a casual barb. Sometimes, he wouldn't acknowledge me at all. I coughed as I walked up the cracking back steps to the house and he made a snarky comment about me quitting smoking.

"I don't smoke anymore. I'm pregnant." There, I'd done it.

"Are you really?" A faint smile crawled across his face, and he quickly moved it aside.

"Yes."

"Well, congratulations, but do you really want to bring a child into this world? It's not the same place as it was when you were little. The planet is so overpopulated, and there are so many kids that need a good home."

"Thanks Dad, we're excited too."

"Just consider adopting before you go getting pregnant again."

I didn't understand how his mind worked. And I wanted to; I really did. Or at one time I did. Now I just braced against what might be coming at any time. I hoped that my turning to stone hadn't hardened the baby in some way, and she understood we had to do that when he came around. Would I teach her the survival techniques or take her from this place so fast that she'd never know it as her home?

Time was drawing to an end; there was no denying that this baby was ready to enter the world. I still tried my best to keep it clinical. I came into each OB-GYN appointment with a list of questions, as though we were working together in a lab and merely discussing the natural progression of mammalian gestation. When I asked if I should take Lamaze classes or some type of birth-preparedness thing where I could be tested on my readiness and feel confident moving forward, he said:

"Are you getting an epidural?"

"Absolutely."

He shrugged, "Then don't bother."

But shouldn't I . . .

It didn't feel right but was easier than going into the *what if* territory of the infinite, universal glory and agony of motherhood. It lay trembling just below the surface of my consciousness but I couldn't burst open in that way.

The feeling of pregnancy "just happening" all over my body was never more acute than when labor began. I could not be mentally present for any of it: the internal exams, the measuring of fluid, the discussions of "incompetent pelvis" and "traumatic for both you and the baby," and even talk that the baby wouldn't fit out at all. I was told that my pubic bone hangs over my birth canal. It was past my due date and the baby had not even dropped. "There is nowhere for her to go," my ob-gyn said. I was convinced that I'd clenched my body for so long that she had no hope of escaping it.

Then I heard, "It's your legal right to choose a caesarean section . . ."

Yes, I could do that. I could make a decision; do something to my body and stop it from doing things to me. I could take control. A decision to intervene surgically would put this thing on my clock and lift the gray mist of the unknown that had settled around me.

But wait . . .

The illusion of control is a powerful thing. It saved me in that moment but then brought me to the point of no return—where I truly knew what it meant to be at the mercy of another human being.

Blue is the return, the ascent. Blue is the sharp reminder, here in the physical, that we are greater than our experience of this place. We remember ourselves within this color—we remember times before and outside of here.

When we finally had a quiet moment in the hospital room, I turned to my husband and said, "If a decision has to be made, choose me. Do you understand? Choose me." He seemed shocked, like he hadn't thought of that possibility, and managed a reply. "Okay . . . if that's what you want."

It was the last bit of control I had to relinquish.

It felt as though years had passed as I was waiting to get into the operating room, but once I was in there, everything moved so quickly. Doctors and residents scrubbing in, anesthesiologists discussing doses and checking lines, hectic cleaning at the back of the room, testing of scales and equipment. I shook with nerves as I hefted my weight up on the plank-like surgical table. The nurse let me look into her eyes and held my arms in a comforting way. Then the pinch of spinal tap and wave of terror, and the cold epidural settled into my limbs with its numbness.

"I am putting the catheter in. Let me know if you feel anything."

"Can you move your legs?"

"We are going to do small tests with the scalpel to see if you are numb yet. Do you feel anything?"

The lower half of my body was the ocean I'd been swallowing, infinite and heavy. I could drag it across land but could not control where it settled. I wondered if that was what mermaids felt when they came ashore.

My husband's smile could be seen all around his face mask. I thought how lucky he was to be removed from the physical realities of having a child. As much as I tried, I couldn't be resentful.

He was so excited, so in love with me, and so in love with what our family was about to become. I wouldn't open myself up to that. Not yet.

The anesthesiologist had a kind face and told me of a medicinal "martini" he would administer as soon as the baby was out. And I was grounded by the knowledge that the pregnancy would be over after my time in this very room, on this very night. Something would end, making room for something to begin.

But my focus still returned to that sheet and the vastness that lay beyond it. Even looking at the top of the doctor's head made me shake with an uncontrollable urge to sneeze and cough at the same time. I believed I could shoot my intestines across the room, or surely burst some necessary capillary.

That is what realization feels like—a pulling. I'd chosen to be powerless after a decade of strangle-holding every ounce of determined self-reliance I had scavenged. And now, the rest of my days could be determined by a roll of the dice. If something were to go terribly wrong, my husband would have the option to choose his nearly born daughter's life over my own. And he would be well within his rights to do so. No one would hate him for it. They would hug him, tell him what a difficult choice he'd made and how at least he has something by which to remember me. This is when my upper body began to quake. I couldn't stop the shaking. I felt the burst of adrenaline from being cut so deeply. Fight or flight is not an option when the lower half of your body is a busted levy. Being a woman opens you up to the world. I felt the room flooding, like the water would never stop pouring out of me because I'd allowed the first cut.

I saw icebergs. I saw glaciers and pristine blue waters with stark white chunks of ice falling—piercing the reflective surface. The sea's surface absorbed the blows and returned to stillness. I felt the chill of nothingness over my skin, jaw trembling. I stayed in this place for as long as I could. I turned my head to the left and held a distant gaze, interacting with no one and nothing. The quiet permeated my consciousness. There were no bodies to contend with, no decisions. Just ice and snow falling into arctic waters with the calmest blues my mind's eye could create. There was strangeness to the silent crashing, a bursting inward and outward at the same time; like being born.

"You will feel a lot of pressure now. This is it, she's almost here." No pressure, no pain, but a cry—a foreign, insistent cry that opened the lungs and burned itself to memory. I didn't understand it or know what to do with it. *That is your child, that is your child, that is your child, feel something.* But I only had medicinal martini haze and confusion. Why would my mind and body allow disassociation to rob me of one of the most precious and important moments of my life?

She was brought to my head. I kissed her face, smiled for a picture with the large blue sheet looming in the background, hiding the earth's waters.

She was here, and I was nailed down to a table. I looked to my husband. "Stay with that baby. Don't take your eyes off of her for a moment." And then they were wheeled out of my life. The doctors sewed the vastness back into my body and brought me into the recovery room.

I would not consciously hold my baby until the next morning, after a tortuous, sleepless night. When she was handed to me, I tried to jump into character, convinced that I would have the same unfortunate nonchalance I had when hearing her first cry. She was crying then, nearly enraged. I took her into my arms and held her against my body and the crying immediately stopped. Recognition.

She knew me. She knew me as her mother. And I knew her then, my body knew her and something kicked in—like the breath of a galloping rhino, powerful, primal, protective, and terrified. It bounded down on me while empowering me, at the same time. And I was very afraid. But I would love that creature enough to make me powerless; neither of us deserved less.

The eternal can live in moments, just as decades of my personal history compressed into small spaces of time when seeing my daughter felt more like remembering her. These moments expanded and contracted for the first three years of her life, as though our present was merely entering and reentering a shared history. But when I went back into my childhood, I went alone and stayed only long enough to gain understanding. Then I ran like hell back to the light—I still run.

i didn't dream
of pregnancy

~ *Tyrese L. Coleman* ~

I'D BREATHLESSLY ARRIVED AT the arcade for the birthday party
of my friend's little boy. Once inside, I sent my kid off into a
jungle gym maze, got a plate of food, and plopped down next to
another girlfriend who was very pregnant. "I'm ready for this
to be over," she said, pulling at her clothes and shifting her weight
in the rigid steel seat. She was cute and flawless. A body-con
maternity dress hugged her perfectly round belly, black hair
pressed straight and slick, no swollen nose or ankles. Pregnancy
looked good on her. But she was clearly uncomfortable, and in
the late-spring Maryland heat, I sympathized.

As if inquiring about a jail sentence, I asked her how much
more time she had. She replied that her caesarean section was
planned for the following week. I immediately became alarmed,
expecting her to follow up by telling me something was not quite
right with the baby. I didn't know anyone who had scheduled a
C-section absent a medical need. She reassured me with a quick
head shake, however. "There's nothing wrong. I wanted one," she
said. If I had just bitten into the hot wing I had left on my plate,

this statement would've definitely left me choking from surprise. This was her first child, and I couldn't believe she was choosing to have a C-section. I had to stop myself from giving her a hug.

She was not like my other friends. I've had many conversations with mothers in our group about my own caesarean section where I've said the same—that I wanted a C-section—even if my twins had not been born prematurely, even if that decision had not been made for me only a few moments before their arrival. Their responses were that they understand why I had one, but, for them, they would never consider having an elective C-section when they could give birth vaginally. They had many reasons: wanting the experience of a traditional childbirth; not wanting to go through what it takes to recover from the operation; wanting, after birth, to focus on their baby and not on themselves.

I get that. I really do. But why do we birthing parents feel we have to sacrifice ourselves and our bodies for the sake of our children? Vaginal labor is not only physical but also symbolic. Even after that first giving up: inception and gestation. A vaginal birth says, "Here, I give myself over to you." Just the beginning of such sacrifices that will happen throughout the course of our lives with our children.

Unpopular opinion number one: The decision to have an elective C-section is an act of empowerment. It means you truly know yourself, what your body can handle, and you shirk the inevitable judgment from people who believe the only legitimate birth experience—whatever that means—involves a vagina. When I heard my girlfriend say she wanted a C-section regardless of her healthy pregnancy and baby—that she wanted this for her very first pregnancy—I nodded emphatically, touched her knee, and said, "Good for you."

We had a long conversation then. She confessed I'd been one of the few people to support her decision. Many had tried to convince her to change her mind, arguing that she would regret not trying for a vaginal birth. They reacted the same when she expressed indifference toward breastfeeding—she would try, but not beat herself up if for some reason it didn't work out. I admired her and her ability not to be persuaded by those trying to impose their own ideas about what a mother should and should not do. A pregnant belly seems to be an invitation for people to share their antiquated, patriarchal notions on pregnancy, birth, and parenting, as if the physical protrusion beyond the boundaries of an average body is a reaching hand asking for some imaginary blessing.

Rarely does this advice consider the needs and desires of the birthing parent. Prenatal and parenting cultures have straddled the hipster movement. Along with craft beers and beards, people are seeking cleaner ways of life, including a return to body-centered birthing and parenting techniques. More women are breastfeeding and letting their babies wean themselves off breast milk and on to food, food made directly in the home by a parent instead of the smelly, soupy, processed goop we were fed. Baby-wearing is ubiquitous, and many women are choosing to have home births, sans an epidural, as a way to connect with their bodies and their babies. As an attempt at what they perceive as an "authentic" birthing experience. This all feels like an endeavor to return to the way our ancestors did things, before the conveniences of drugs and preservatives and everything else that makes life much easier to live. It reminds me of that scene from *Apocalypto* where Jaguar Paw's wife, Seven, gives birth to their baby while trapped inside a muddy and flooding pit cave. Now, *she* would have full bragging rights in the mommy wars for centuries.

Most actively seeking these natural courses are first-time parents. It makes sense that when you are having your first child you would want to do what you perceive is right and best from as early on as possible. But, how do you know what's right and what's best?

Partly by a desire to do the opposite of what our parents did. This desire is subconscious, ingrained in the ways we survive as a species. By outdoing the group before ours, we ensure our own longevity, generation after generation. We may all be in competition with our peers for jobs or romantic partners, but in terms of our lives and legacies, we compete with our parents. This is why I decided to go to law school; why I decided to get married before having children; why I decided to do what I could to outearn my mother and father—the ingrained need to do better than they did.

And what did our parents do in terms of rearing this era of new and natural parents? They gave us chemically-enriched formula. They had "easy," highly-medicated labors. They used non-biodegradable disposable diapers. I know the benefits of breast milk, of not overmedicating, of saving the earth. But I also believe that some of the machinations of holistic parenting belie an insecurity, a distrust of our parents or a fear of becoming them. Foregoing the convenience of formula, the painlessness of an epidural, or the simplicity of disposable diapers means more effort and more stress for new parents. We are masochistic, thinking that the more we put on ourselves the more credit we deserve, and the more *real* we are. This is less about what is best for the child, and even less about what is best for the parents, especially the one who gives birth. Having a child doesn't have to be this hard.

Here is my second unpopular opinion: Childbirth is trauma. Consider the physicality of it. There is a foreign being inside of you, a growth, a parasite, that needs to get out. It convulses and swells. It forces you open from the inside, using its head or feet, the strongest parts of any body, to make its own way, despite the already determined curvature and anatomy of its host, prying that host apart, splitting her in the middle. Childbirth rips you apart. Excuse me if I am a traitor to my generation, but I am not into torturing myself. I have never wanted that. I have never wanted to give birth that way. And although I did not have the choice at the time, if I did, I would still have decided to have a C-section.

I didn't dream of pregnancy. I was never one of those little girls who placed a pillow down the front of her pants, a hand on her hip or back, waddling around and pretending to carry twins. I was the child who turned that pillow around and stuffed it down the back of her pants—the old lady with a big butt. I mothered my dolls, combed their hair and dressed them, without considering how they may have arrived if they were real-life Baby Alives.

Not until I was old enough to feel the weight of death squatting on my chest, did children become a part of my life plan. I harbor a debilitating fear of dying. It keeps me awake at night. And during one of those sleepless evenings, when anxiety and fear pressed down on me, I thought: What if I have a child. And the weight eased. Ralph Waldo Emerson wrote, "It is the secret of the world that all things subsist and do not die, but retire a little from sight and afterwards return again." And each night I felt the pressure, I soothed myself by thinking of my future children, of what would subsist of me.

This desire for a legacy, a way to live further, even when I am gone, began to manifest in other, more nurturing ways. I would see children at the store or mall or in my neighborhood, and find that I wanted to hold them, that I desperately wanted to feel the weight of a baby on my chest instead of fear. It became a yearning, and I ached at the sight of a baby.

I longed for children, but, to be clear, I did not long to be pregnant. Pregnancy was only a means to an end.

I am ashamed to admit how ignorant I was about the concept of birth when I was pregnant. I grew up in the South, where public schools gave a basic "Family Health" education that involved gender-segregated classrooms and colorful posters of the female reproductive system. I knew about uteruses and cervixes and vulvas. Those posters showed me the position a baby takes in the womb at different stages of pregnancy, but never exactly what happened when the baby comes out.

I wasn't completely ignorant about the functioning of my own equipment. Some women don't even know what their vagina looks like. I disposed of that cliché early on, often staring at it in the dresser mirror that faced my bed as a kid. Even after examining it for most of my life, there is always a spark of surprise by its sight. But, honestly, even if I hadn't looked, I would still know my body. I know it inside and out. There is scar tissue. And even when we can't see them, we know our scars, and we know the anatomy of our wounds.

It wasn't until I was pregnant that I became curious about what happens to a woman's body during childbirth. It was early on—it had to be. I had my twins at twenty-five weeks. I was on modified bed rest after a cerclage at twenty-two weeks, watching Discovery Health. Back-to-back episodes of *A Birth Story* made me curious, and I googled "birth video." I watched in silence as the baby's head broke through, anxiety radiating through me along with that pulsing vulva across the small, palm-sized screen of my phone. The baby's head, a diamond-shaped sliver of black slickened hair, peeked through, then burst out. I squeezed my legs in response to the scene, buried my face into my pillow. That video solidified what had been only a subconscious inkling: I did not want to give birth vaginally. I knew this all along, but the video allowed me to confront the concept of birth in a way I had not before.

I don't know when the idea of not having a vaginal birth manifested. Maybe it was as early as the day we found out I was having twins. After trying to conceive for more than a year, my husband and I decided to get help at a fertility clinic. The walls of every fertility clinic are lined with postcards, holiday cards, family portraits of successful clients—free advertising. Most of the families have multiples, and, indeed, on the very first visit, our doctor informed us that the likelihood of having a multiples pregnancy was much higher than it would be if we conceived without medical assistance. Any amount of research into multiple pregnancies will tell you that there is a greater chance of having a caesarean section and that they result in higher instances of prematurity. That conversation occurred between six and eight weeks, when the decision to have a C-section was merely a grain of thought, as tiny as the babies inside me. It would eventually work itself into a pearl.

Or maybe it was before that, before I got pregnant. Maybe I made the decision to never have a vaginal birth during those long months of injecting myself with hormones, digesting multiple pills, or having uninspired, timed *intercourse* that felt as lifeless and clinical as the word. Because back then, the thought of all of that work, and of me—actually pregnant—seemed like such a distant and ridiculous dream, that I never processed the possibility of having a baby, let alone two.

But now, I surmise it was well before that. Well before I met my husband. Before I met my ex-boyfriend, a man who, despite my complaints of pain during sex, despite my biological response of unwanting—the lack of any natural lubrication—continued to pound into my body as if he felt that he could imprint his likeness on a child by forcing his entire body into my vagina. Before that violation created a four-inch tear right there, right where a baby comes from, for which I needed emergency surgery. Before it burned with pain to have him inside me, never mind a baby coming out of me. Before he called to check on me after the procedure, but never apologized.

But, you know, it could've been even before that. I could've decided that I never wanted to have a vaginal birth back when the violations to my body were more subtle, hidden because it appeared as though I sought them out. Violations that involved multiple partners, and strangers, and too much drinking. Violations I don't remember; violations I did not want. Violations I thought were empowering, but instead were coping mechanisms resulting from other violations. My body is worn. The wounds still rigid with the atrophy of recent violence. Forgive me for not wanting to endure more. Forgive me for not wanting to associate my children with the continued violation of my body.

Or maybe, I made this decision even further back. Back when I was a nine-year-old, and had my first period. Back when I was the only girl in elementary school carrying maxi pads in her purse. Or back when I went through early puberty, my breasts forming so quickly that by the age of seven I needed a bra. Back when old men put me on their lap and bounced me up and down, their hard, bony knees jabbing me in that spot where the world says that only my husband and my children should come near. Or when my mother's boyfriend touched me there in the middle of the night. Back when I was five and had to force his hands off me, back to that very first violation, that very first time someone split me open and ripped me apart.

I could not bear it, despite wanting to bear them.

We get over the trauma. Women are boomerangs. We are stretchy silly putty made of reforming adaptable tissue that stretches us to its limits. Our bellies stretch, our vaginas stretch, our breasts stretch, and then, once pulled to the extreme, pulled beyond recognition, our bodies return to us. I am confident that I would've gotten over the pain of a vaginal birth. But why should I have to?

Does this make me selfish? Yes, it does. Our innate human instinct of survival, those electric impulses in our nervous system that force us awake when we suddenly stop breathing while sleeping or make us fight against drowning still function despite pregnancy, despite having children. Self-preservation is the reason we have children. It is the reason why I sleep better knowing they are here, that they will out-survive me and, one day, outearn, outdo me.

scars of life

An Adoptee's Meditation on
Her C-Section and Hysterectomy

∽ *SooJin Pate* ∾

I CAN'T REMEMBER a time when I didn't want to have a baby. At five years old, I walked around with all manner of stuffed animals under my shirt—bears, bunnies, frogs, and puppies. When it was time for them to be born, I put my hand under my shirt and pulled them out. I patted their backs to make sure they cried. After I heard the yelp that came from their first breath, I lifted my shirt and put their mouth on my pin-drop of a nipple so they could have their first meal. Then I would sing them a song, like my umma did when I sucked in her goodness. But my umma, my mom, was no longer with me. So I would reenact this memory of breastfeeding, over and over again, as a way to feel close to her.

I was taken from my umma when I was five years old. Under Confucian family law at that time in South Korea, a woman had very few rights—especially if she was a divorcee or a widow. My umma was both. My umma had divorced my appa (father) in the summer. They reconciled and came back together in the fall. By winter, my appa died suddenly in an accident. They never legally remarried, so everything she had became the property of my father's family—including her children. My uncle, my father's brother, promised to take care of us. Instead, he put us up for adoption—behind her back—in exchange for money.

My umma only consented to signing the papers that terminated her parental rights because the adoption agency promised that she could see us one more time: She could take us to the airport. Inside the concrete corridor of Kimpo airport, I was stripped from her arms by a white man. No cops were called. No arrests were made. No, this taking away was totally legal. The white man was an escort hired by Lutheran Social Services, the adoption agency that coordinated the relocation of me and my younger sister from the Park family in Seoul, South Korea, to the Link family in Fairmont, Minnesota.

I cried on the plane from Seoul to Portland, and to our final stop in Minneapolis. I cried during the two-and-a-half-hour drive from Minneapolis to Fairmont, a small southern Minnesota town. My arrival to the United States was full of trauma, loss, and pain. As a way to comfort myself, I recollected memories of my umma breastfeeding me or singing to me as I lay on her lap. I returned to these scenes over and over again—so much so that they would come alive in my dreams. In my dream space, I was able to find my way back to Korea, return home to my umma. Only upon waking did I realize that it was only a dream. So I would try to animate my dreams in the daytime through dramatic play. I tried to conjure up the motherlove I so desperately missed in my new adoptive family, even if it meant reversing the roles: me as the mother, and my stuffed animal as the child.

As I grew into adulthood, the concept of becoming a mother became less about comforting myself and more about healing the forced mother-daughter separation that took place via my adoption. I wanted the opportunity to correct a horrible wrong; I wanted a second chance to experience the mother-daughter bond that was cut short when I was five years old. But I wanted to do it right. First, I needed a stable career. Then, I wanted to find the right partner. But most importantly, I wanted to heal the trauma of adoption so that I wouldn't pass that trauma onto my child. When I moved to the Twin Cities to attend college after I graduated from high school, I found myself a good therapist and did the emotional and spiritual excavation necessary to do just that.

~

I had just started graduate school, the first step to becoming a professor of race and ethnic studies. My biological clock was ticking louder than ever, when I received news after a routine pap smear that I had adenocarcinoma in situ of the cervix. This was the same exact diagnosis that Henrietta Lacks received—the woman now famous for her immortal cells. I was in my early twenties. My oncologist-gynecologist said it was very rare for someone so young to receive such a diagnosis. I couldn't get past the *carcinoma* part of what he said. Did I have cancer? My doctor assured me that I didn't have cancer; however, he did find precancerous cells that could eventually lead to cancer. And if they did turn cancerous, the cancer would most certainly be advanced because this particular type was hard to detect (since it developed in the deeper, glandular section of the cervix), and symptoms only appeared when it was too late. The recommended treatment: a total hysterectomy.

Back in 1951 when Lacks received the same diagnosis, a total hysterectomy was considered too invasive and extreme. But it would have saved her life. It is now considered standard protocol; however, getting a hysterectomy was out of the question for me because I wanted to have a child. Desperately. I needed to have a daughter—to heal and mend my childhood past. I asked my doctor if there was an alternative treatment that could allow me to have a baby. There was.

In an effort to preserve my ability to bear a child, I underwent a conization to remove a portion of my cervix that was affected with precancerous cells. In addition, I went in for a routine pap smear every six months. I did this during the first few years of my PhD program until I completed my coursework and exams. As a gift to myself for becoming ABD (all but dissertation), I told my husband, "It's time for us to make a baby now." And we did.

My first trimester was filled with all the clichéd markers of pregnancy: throwing up like clockwork twice a day—once in the morning and once at night, craving weird combinations of food, and being sickened by food and smells that I typically loved. But on the first day of my second trimester, everything changed. All the nausea and sensitivity to food and smells went away. And I felt like superwoman. I felt powerful, luscious, vibrant, and ripe. I had never felt so sexy and strong in my entire life.

I wanted the conditions in which my daughter entered the world to be at their most optimal and pure (meaning, not medically invasive). That's why I decided to have a natural birth. I had read that medicines like Pitocin and epidurals increased the chances of having a C-section. That was the last thing I wanted. The thought of having a C-section terrified me. It seemed unnatural. I had friends who opted to have a C-section over a vaginal birth because they could schedule the delivery at a time that was most convenient for them. They loved the convenience of it. Not me. I welcomed the surprise of my daughter choosing to come out when she was ready. And I wanted my daughter to come *through* me—not to be plucked out from some man-made surgical incision.

This process of coming *through* me was especially significant because of my history as a transracial adoptee. For many

transracial and transnational adoptees, the desire to have someone in your family who looks like you is a common one. This
yearning for a mirror reflection is a natural stage of childhood;
however, because most adoptees from Africa, Asia, and South
America are adopted by white Americans who live in all-white
communities, this desire for a mirror is rarely ever fulfilled. That's
why having a baby has an additional layer of meaning for many
adoptees: it's our way of providing ourselves with our own mirror.
"Having a baby is the only way I could have someone in my family
who looked like me," a friend once shared with me. Other friends
have expressed this sentiment: "I've never met anyone who was
biologically related to me until my [daughter or son] was born."

For me, the process of a vaginal birth made this biological
connection between me and my child even more visceral and
intimate. I couldn't wait for the moment when I could see her tuft
of black hair peek through between my legs. I couldn't wait to
hear the doctor say, "Almost there! Just one more push!" And I
couldn't wait to feel the sensation of my baby girl sliding out of
me. Hearing the stories of my friends who had undergone natural
births, I had romanticized the whole scene in my head. I wanted
to experience all these things—to feel every sensation—so I
drafted a birth plan and hired a doula in the hopes that writing
down my intentions would make it so.

My first and most important lesson regarding parenthood came
on the day when my birth plan fell apart. I woke up one morning
with my panties slightly wet. Not sure if my water was about to
break, I decided to go to the hospital. I was leaking amniotic fluid,
but there were no signs that my water was about to break; the
nurses, however, didn't want to send me home, so they checked me
into the hospital. Knowing that I wanted a natural birth, they
waited to see if my body would naturally progress without the

intervention of medicine. Several hours went by and they decided to induce me with Pitocin for fear of infection setting in.

Violating the first item listed in my birth plan—no medication—had a domino effect that led to the breaching of every single item on my birth plan. (In hindsight, my birth plan falling apart was probably the most effective induction into parenthood I could have had.) I was in labor for over thirty hours and pushed for another four—two hours longer than the ob-gyn was comfortable with—because I just wanted at least one thing on my birth plan to go right: the ability to give birth to my baby vaginally. But my daughter's body got stuck in the birth canal at a 10-to-4 o'clock position. No longer comfortable with the situation, the ob-gyn ordered an emergency C-section. I felt demoralized. This was the thing that I feared the most, the one thing that I didn't want to happen. No matter how hard I tried to prevent this very thing from happening, there was no way around it. And so, I cried. My ob-gyn reminded me that delivering a healthy baby and keeping me safe were her priorities. She continued by explaining that once my baby was born, it wouldn't matter how she came out because the joy of holding her in my arms would outweigh the method in which she was delivered.

My ob-gyn was right. Having a healthy baby in my arms made the fact that my birth plan went to shit quite insignificant.

～

My daughter was three years old when I received my first abnormal pap smear since the conization procedure that had removed the precancerous area of my cervix. Even before I received the lab results, I knew that this particular exam would return abnormal results because I had been warned in my dreams. Several months prior to my bi-monthly checkup, I started dreaming that I was dying of cervical cancer. These dreams were so frequent and so visceral that I said to my husband nonchalantly after dinner one night, "I've been having visions of my death almost every night. I know how I'm going to die. I'm going to die of cervical cancer." So when my gynecologist oncologist told me that my pap smear was abnormal and that I should get that hysterectomy that he recommended years ago, I wasn't surprised. I knew what needed to be done, but I didn't want to undergo the procedure out of fear. I wanted the surgery because I was ready—not because I was afraid to die. At that point, I wasn't quite sure if I wanted more children. My daughter had been asking for a little brother or sister. Other friends and family members encouraged me to have at least one more—for the sake of my daughter. "You don't want her to be the only child, do you? Think about how lonely she'll be. Think about how all the responsibility will rest on her shoulders if you or your husband get sick," they'd say. These questions posed by my loved ones made me wonder if I should try to get pregnant one more time, while I still had the chance. I asked my doctor if I could have a little more time to think about the timing of my surgery, and he agreed. I eventually decided against having another child and, finally, got the total hysterectomy.

Because it was a total hysterectomy, my doctor suggested that three to four weeks recovery time was optimal. But women usually took two weeks off from work. I didn't have enough paid time off or vacation hours to take a full two weeks, so I ended up taking one week off and working the second week from home.

I went home with the following doctor's orders: Rest. Rest. Rest. Don't lift anything over five-to-ten pounds. Take pain medication, as needed. And listen to your body. I did just that: I listened to my body, and it told me to sleep. I slept for nearly three days straight, only waking up long enough to take my medication and go to the bathroom. The side effects from anesthesia and pain medication made me groggy and nauseous. I could barely keep my eyes open or eat during those first three days. By the end of the first week, I wasn't as fatigued as I had been; however, I still had a lot of pain when walking, standing, or sitting, and when I had to get up and down from the couch or bed or toilet. Working from home that second week of recovery was difficult. Sitting upright with a computer aggravated my abdominal area. But it was better than having to make the hour-long, roundtrip commute and sitting at a desk for eight hours straight.

During recovery, I couldn't help but think of the last time I had surgery—when I had my C-section. The surgeries were similar in that the incisions were in the same area. The pain I experienced was similar, too, especially when I tried to sit, stand, or walk. But the recoveries were completely different. I remembered that the second day after my C-section, I was walking around the hospital room, holding my seven-pound baby. Being on my feet and taking care of a brand new baby seemed unthinkable as I lay on the couch recuperating from my hysterectomy. But I did it, And it was painful. Since I was nursing, I didn't take pain medication. Bathing my daughter, changing her diaper, dressing her— all the usual duties that came with taking care of a newborn—were things I did four days after I returned home from my C-section.

I remember having to hunch forward to hold my daughter, six months after the procedure, because the strain of standing and walking was too painful. It took a full year before I could sit or stand without pain shooting from my midsection. In contrast, five weeks after my hysterectomy, I was running around Bde Maka Ska, the lake near my house. What was the difference? I recovered so much faster after my hysterectomy than after my C-section because of the care and treatment I received post-operation. When I was discharged from my C-section, the instructions from my doctor were all about my baby. There was little said about the fact that I had undergone major surgery. It was as if I hadn't had surgery at all; I simply delivered a baby and my only responsibility was to take care of that baby. I came home on a Saturday and had the weekend with my husband before he was off to work on Monday. After that, it was just me and my newborn daughter.

After my hysterectomy, I had clear instructions from my doctor to focus on my recovery. My sister stayed with me those two weeks and waited on me, hand and foot. She kept track of when and how much medicine I needed to take. She helped me get up to go to the bathroom. Her body acted as a cane, assisting me every time I needed to walk from point A to point B. No wonder I recovered so much more quickly: I was treated by my doctors, my family who took care of me, and my friends who dropped off food and visited—as if I'd had surgery. The focus was on my recovery. In contrast, my C-section—because it was simply a means to deliver my baby—was dislodged from the context of surgery and replaced by the celebratory moment of the birth of a healthy baby girl. The excitement of birth far outweighed the fact of surgery, so the focus was on the new baby, instead of the recovering mother.

Before having my baby, I was afraid of having a C-section because it was "unnatural" and seemed antithetical to the "natural" process of a vaginal birth. I wanted the imprint of the medical establishment to be as small as possible when it came to the birth of my child. That's why I hired a doula—to increase the chances of a natural birth and decrease the chances of getting a C-section.

What everyone failed to point out—including the general public, the medical establishment, and my friends who chose to have a C-section—is that it is major surgery. No one talks about C-sections as surgery. They talk about it as if it's just another way—albeit more *convenient* way—of giving birth.

Decontextualizing a C-section as surgery and recontextualizing it as an alternative to vaginal birth is a huge disservice to the mother, especially a first-timer. There is an unspoken expectation that the mother be "up and at 'em" upon giving birth, and it's not realistic. Unlike my post-operation instructions after my hysterectomy, I received no order of bed rest or to stay off my feet, let alone not to carry anything over five to ten pounds. Even with maternity leave, there was no period of recovery allotted to me. No wonder my recovery time exponentially multiplied. It took me over a year to be able to take a three-mile run after my C-section. It took me just five weeks to run that same distance post-hysterectomy. I was allotted the time and space to recover—I was treated as if I had undergone major surgery.

~

When my daughter was born, I craned my head to look past the curtain separating my chest from my abdomen so I could see her face. I longed to see her face. I wanted to see what parts of me made it into her. During the first few months of her life, I studied her face diligently. As a transracial and transnational adoptee, it was thrilling to be able to look into her eyes and see myself in her eyebrows, cheeks, and lips. Now that my daughter is older, I'm taken aback by what I don't see. What's absent when I peer into her sparkling onyx eyes, is the sadness that comes from forced, premature separation of a parent and child. She will never know the pain that comes from being stripped from my arms.

One night, as I tucked her into bed, my daughter gently traced the line of my C-section with her finger and said—more to herself than to me—"This is where I came from."

"Yes, you came out of mama's tummy right here," I replied, retracing the scar with my fingers. "I pushed and pushed and tried with all my might so that you could come through me, but your head got stuck on the way out, so they had to cut you out instead."

This is a conversation my daughter and I have had several times over the years. From time to time, she will ask me to tell her about when she was a baby. Tracing my C-section scar has become a ritual of sorts whenever I recount her birth story. I think she likes to hear about the time she was born because it reminds her that she was wanted—has always been wanted—because I worked so hard to bring her into the world (and wished for her long before she came). My C-section scar serves as a marker of that labor, of that wish. As a result, we both look at it and touch it, lovingly.

High above my C-section scar now sits the scar from my hysterectomy. One scar gave me my heart's desire. The other ensures that my life isn't snuffed out prematurely by cancer so I can nurture that heart's desire for as long as possible. In this way, both cuts gave life. While the first cut gave life to my daughter, the second cut gave *me* life. My daughter and I share the same lifeline and it is recorded—hardcoded as scar tissue—on my belly.

notes from the lying-in hospital

∿ *Nicole Cooley* ⌒

I'LL LEARN THIS LATER: The original purpose of a C-section is to remove a baby from a dead or dying mother to save the baby.

And if the baby can't be saved, the purpose of a C-section is to ensure that the dead baby and the dead mother could be buried separately.

∿

Now the irises rage light, spiked tongues
at my hospital window—

How I would like to just unravel.

Through glass, cut leaves curl like fingers
in my throat.

How I once wished to take myself apart.

∿

Once upon a time, in the other story, there was a woman, a not-yet mother. She was pregnant and sat at the window, watching a garden that did not belong to her. The garden full of rampion *so fresh and green that she longed for it.* She wanted that green. She wished for handful after handful of the flowering scab that grew in the garden next door.

~

All my life, I've believed I'll die in childbirth, though there is no reason at all for me to think this. As a child, as a teenager, and well into my thirties, I convinced myself that birth is inextricable from death: that my giving birth will lead to my death.

~

At home, weeks after the birth, the scar is a half-moon, a low-lying smile. Red line snaking on my skin, thinner than I thought yet more painful. Unless I study myself closely in a mirror, I can't see the site of the incision. The scar is less dramatic than I imagine. It's a line erasing what happened with my daughter's birth.

My baby girl is more beautiful than I could have imagined: dark shining eyes, arms and legs pumping in pleasure when she sees me enter the room. I pick her up and her face turns against my shoulder, her small arms reach over mine.

The scar. The girl.

I've been told over and over that one is supposed to cancel the other out. I've been told that all that matters is the outcome of the birth.

Yet I've also been told that my baby's ability to love me has been compromised by her birth. I've been told her birth was not natural. I've been told I could have done so much to prevent what happened to me. I've been told I should have had a better birth plan. I've been told I should have asserted myself more with my doctors. I've been told my emergency C-section was my fault.

A hundred years ago my daughter and I would both be dead.

These are the images, but most people would rather not hear the story.

~

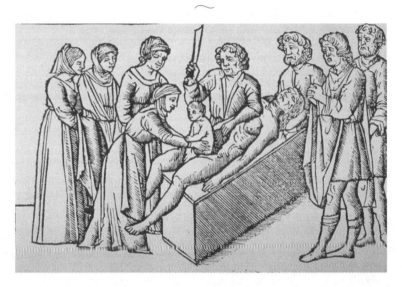

Caesarean section reproduction. Based on Suetonius' *Lives of the Twelve Caesars* woodcut, 1506.

~

In the 1799 Lying-In Hospital, first on Broome Street, now part of the old stone building at New York Hospital, my husband and I have my twenty-week sonogram. Strange to enter a two-hundred-year-old hospital that resembles a cathedral for cutting edge technological medical tests.

After, my husband and I wait in the hallway for our results. On a wooden bench, we wait, and with every minute that passes we know something is wrong.

At last, the doctor calls us into his office. "The sonogram picked something up. There's a calcium deposit on one of the four chambers of the fetus' heart. It has a link to Down syndrome and other problems. We think that you should know that further testing will be required immediately."

I say nothing. I only stare, absurdly, at an article on his desk that the doctor submitted to *Obstetrics and Gynecology*. I keep my eyes focused on the rejection letter. I can relate to it, I think, with my own submissions and rejections of my poems. I wonder how he felt when his article was rejected. Considering that is easier than listening to what the doctor has to say.

⁓

The history of cesarean section can be understood best in the broader context of the history of childbirth and general medicine histories that also have been characterized by dramatic changes. Many of the earliest successful cesarean sections took place in remote rural areas lacking in medical staff and facilities. . . . These operations were performed on kitchen tables and beds.

⁓

Woodcuts: the mother's body splayed open on a table. I turn the pages of the book slowly and I can't stop looking.

⁓

In the other story, the woman's husband became a thief. She *pined away*. She said she *would die* if he could not bring her the rampion, and so he climbed the high wall, slipped into the enchantress's garden, ripped leaves from stalks, dug up the plant's long roots that leaked milky liquid all over his hands.

This plant, this herb, this bitter metallic taste that split her tongue like a knife—the woman could not get enough of it.

⁓

All my life I've believed that I'll die in childbirth, and once I'm pregnant no one can convince me this is not true, although I'm planning to give birth to my child in New York City, at a top hospital, in the twenty-first century. Nevertheless, throughout my pregnancy, I am convinced I'll die when my daughter is born. I'll exchange my life with hers, and I feel oddly at peace with this equivalence.

I plan to write letters to my unborn daughter, to make a memory box in advance of her birth so she will have something of me to hold on to. I never tell my husband this. I'll assemble the artifacts in secret.

⁓

Yet, the early history of cesarean section remains shrouded in myth and is of dubious accuracy. Even the origin of "cesarean" has apparently been distorted over time. It is commonly believed to be derived from the surgical birth of Julius Caesar, however this seems unlikely since his mother Aurelia is reputed to have lived to hear of her son's invasion of Britain. At that time the procedure was performed only when the mother was dead or dying, as an attempt to save the child for a state wishing to increase its population. Roman law under Caesar decreed that all women who were so fated by childbirth must be cut open; hence, cesarean. Other possible Latin origins include the verb "caedare," meaning to cut, and the term "caesones" that was applied to infants born by postmortem operations.

⁓

I would like to unravel, but I won't.

Because the afternoon at the Lying-In Hospital is just the beginning, the first of the medical tests that will be insisted upon: needles, blood tests, liquids to drink, measurements of tissue and bone. Over and over again, I'm told there is something terribly wrong with my baby and with me. Yet each test is negative. And there are many. I try to refuse them. An HIV test: "If you won't do it now, we will have to stick the baby. It's the New York State Law!" A strep test where I am told I carry a virus potentially fatal to my baby so I'll be chained to an antibiotic drip for the entire birth. Amniocentesis—a needle wicks yellow fluid from my abdomen, my husband looks away, and I watch with a horrid fascination.

I believe I'll die in childbirth. The first C-sections were performed on dead or dying women, a surgical birth to save a fetus because the mother would not survive. C-sections to preserve the life of the mother only were performed in the late nineteenth century until the present. I picture my own dead body, a wound pinned shut with silver stitches, a newborn baby I will never see.

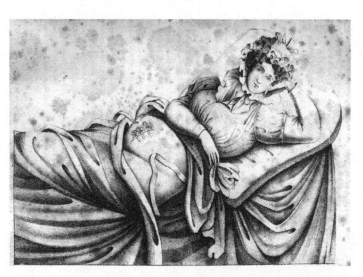

A caesarean patient prior to dressing the wound. From Edward Siebold, *Abbildungen aus dem gesammtgebiete der theoretisch-praktischen geburtshülfe*, 1829.

~

In the story, when the enchantress finds the husband stealing from her garden she is furious. She declares, *I will allow you to take as much rampion as you will, only I make one condition, you must give me the child your wife will bring into the world.* And the pregnant woman makes this promise.

What kind of mother would agree?

~

Perhaps the first written record we have of a mother and baby surviving a cesarean section comes from Switzerland in 1500, when a sow-gelder, Jacob Nufer, performed the operation on his wife. After several days in labor and help from thirteen midwives, the woman was unable to deliver her baby. Her desperate husband eventually gained permission from the local authorities to attempt a cesarean. The mother lived and subsequently gave birth normally to five children, including twins.

~

I want too much. I want all the wrong things. The first hint of the curse that is my pregnancy is the nausea. All day and night, unceasing, like a punishment.

The OB won't give me the real drugs I want, so I take Tums every day. Sweet, chalky, the size of a dime: I grow to like, even love the taste of this medicine. I chew spearmint gum like a teenager. I buy seasickness wristbands. I shred slices of raw ginger between my teeth.

Then, the headaches begin. Someone is drilling, drilling inside my head. Lights flash in my eyes continually when I try to read, the page a blur of silver streaks.

All I can think of is failure: I want the baby, but I hate being pregnant and there's something wrong with me for hating the pregnancy.

I'm told by an uncle, casually, in a phone conversation, that my feeling unwell clearly shows that I don't actually want to be a mother at all.

⁓

As a serious abdominal operation, the development of cesarean section both sustained and reflected changes within general surgery. In the early 1800s, when surgery still relied on age-old techniques, its practitioners were dreaded and viewed by the public as little better than barbers, butchers, and tooth pullers.

⁓

Already I know I'm that bad mother, throat stuffed with dust, mouth a blistering ache, promising anything, forgetting the baby swimming inside me, baby the size of a fist, baby taking root.

⁓

Finally, three days past my due date, when my water breaks at home, I refuse to stay in our apartment, which is what we've been told to do. I refuse to let my husband time contractions. Instead, we drive to the hospital in Manhattan and I inform the staff we are not returning home over the Queensboro Bridge. *We need a room immediately.* The nurses are annoyed, but I insist. It will turn out to be the only time during my entire pregnancy when I'm listened to.

The birthing room where I will not give birth resembles a bland hotel. A Jim Dine print of a red heart is nailed to the wall across from the bed. I will myself to remember it because I want that image to be inextricably connected to my daughter's arrival. *How well-chosen, how appropriate!* I tell my husband; someone must have carefully considered which pictures would look best on the labor floor. I imagine the story I will tell my daughter, later, about this image.

Because, all evidence from the last nine months to the contrary, I believe that her birth will be the kind of story I will want to tell.

My water has broken but nothing is beginning. The nurses who did not want me here are silent and curt, a few hours in. Straps circling my stomach, hooked up to monitors that resound the baby's heartbeat through the room, in piped-in, too-loud stereo, I'm given Cervadil, a gel attached to a string that "will open the cervix to jump-start labor."

Of course, nothing jump-starts. The Cervadil fails. One in a series of what would feel like small, personal failures, leading me down a road I don't want to be on, a road I always knew I would be on. The road leads to Stadol, a narcotic, and then Pitocin, to start labor in earnest, then an epidural.

～

My husband tries to make me laugh by taking pictures, photographs I know never to look at later, of me lying in the bed, immobilized, hooked up to tubes and wires. "I look like a transplant patient," I say, as if that is funny at all.

～

Wanting too much, the other mother drops out of the fairy tale—she has traded her daughter for her other desire. For her selfishness, the enchantress takes her daughter, names her Rapunzel after the rampion, and locks her up in a tower alone. The bad mother pines away with desire, without her daughter now.

～

Poet Alicia Ostriker, in one of her essays on motherhood, writes about feeling like an Olympic athlete, a heroine, a marathon runner, when she was in labor. I think of her essay, which I've long admired, as I breathe in the plastic shell of the oxygen mask a nurse has strapped on my face *because you are not giving the baby enough oxygen.*

Hours into labor, I already know I am the furthest thing from heroic and the birth is not athletic at all.

⁓

The heartbeat resounds through the room. The blue screen beeps. A red line streams across the monitor like a vein. I breathe into my mask and pain shatters my ribcage. Pain ruins each vertebrae of my backbone, drives my bones to dust. Yet nothing is beginning.

⁓

The operation originated from attempts to save the soul, if not the life, of a fetus whose mother was dead or dying. Since ancient times, however, there have been occasional efforts to save the mother, and during the nineteenth century, systematic improvement of cesarean section techniques eventually led to lower mortality for women and their fetuses. Increasingly the operation was performed in cases where the mother's health was considered endangered, in addition to those in which her life was immediately at stake. Finally, in the late twentieth century, in mainstream Western medical society the fetus has become the primary patient once labor has commenced.

⁓

The baby's head is slightly turned, the baby is larger than expected, the baby now is in *visible distress.*

When I hear the doctor say, "There are many different ways to give birth, Nicole," I know this sentence is what she was taught to say in medical school when everything is about to go wrong.

I hear it, and I think, who taught you that? How, I think, could that be revised to be said better?

A catheter is jammed between my legs, a new oxygen cannula inserted in my nose, my body is rolled onto a rubber sheet, the corners lifted, I'm told to cross my arms over my chest and I know that it has finally happened, what I've always known will happen when I give birth: now I'm actually dead.

In the operating room, arms strapped down in a mock-crucifixion pose, I want to ask for my husband, but I'm unable to speak. I don't know where he is.

Where is the baby?

There is no space between us: body caught in my body—

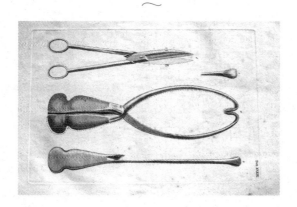

Destructive scissors and crotchets. From William Smellie's
A Sett of Anatomical Tables, 1754.

I can't speak but I'm trying to tell the operating room staff—the room is full of people, blue-gowned so I can't discern identities— that I feel enormous pain when my abdomen is touched. That I know I'll feel the entire operation, that someone must let me up, untie my hands, get me out of the room.

The truth is that I don't feel the surgery at all. Only a slight pressure. Toward the end, an odd ruffling of hands inside my body, near my lungs. The surgical team is moving around too high inside my body. I try to picture the drawings of the pregnant body from the useless Lamaze class handouts. Later, I will be told that my daughter never dropped down into my pelvis.

Then the baby is here. She's shown to us, suspended above my head, and she is large, but, I don't feel the promised surge of emotion—gratitude and love and joy. I just think, *Oh, okay, that's the baby*, and *now it's okay if I am dead*.

⁓

The voice: *There are many different ways to give birth.*

⁓

Freezing and shaking in Recovery: *I will never do this again*, I tell my husband. He says nothing, tightens the folds of the heated blanket on my legs.

⁓

Hours later, we're checked into a hospital room and no one has brought us our baby.

Our baby is missing. No one seems to know where she is.

Maybe, I think, I didn't give birth to an actual baby. Maybe I simply had a bloody and terrible operation and doctors took something else out of my body, something they won't ever return to me now.

Or maybe I've done something so terrible that I will never see my baby again.

At 9:30 PM, two neonatologists, with no baby, come into the room, stand together at the edge of my bed, and tell us they think our baby very likely has a severe brain defect, and would we sign

this clipboard of forms so she can have an MRI and be sedated?
Our baby who is six hours old.

⁓

Once upon a time, in that story, the unborn baby was promised
away. Once upon a time, a daughter grew up without her mother.
Once upon a time, a bad mother devoured and devoured and now
she will never hold her daughter.

⁓

Now all is slow motion: Across from my bed is a large black and
white clock, the kind in a grade school classroom, and we watch
the time drag. I vomit and doze and beg the nurse for relief from
nausea and pain until she gives me a shot. My husband cries in the
bathroom so I won't know, but I know. Until hours later when the
baby is wheeled back in, and we're told her brain is perfect and
intact. *False alarm. Just a scare.* The older neonatologist smiles at us.
Everyone is casual. Meanwhile we hug and hug the baby. We call
her by her name for the first time because we believe, at last, that
she will stay. We decide her middle name will be Iris, after my
favorite flower. She's finally ours and we hold her all night. We
can't bear to ever again put her down, alone in her glass bassinet.

⁓

Is it the curse, or is it because of my C-section that two days later
my baby is taken away, again for hours, this time for tests on her
heart? Is it because of my C-section that my three-day-old baby is
given an EKG, then an echocardiogram? Is it because of my
C-section that I sit in the hall with my IV pole, praying and begging and uselessly bartering, waiting for her to be wheeled out of
the Cardiac Testing Unit?

Sitting in the hall in my hospital bathrobe and awful gray socks to prevent me from slipping, tethered to my IV, I make trade-offs: I'll be less obsessed by my job, I'll care less about teaching, I'll be a nicer person if she can just be saved. And again, she is returned to us, healthy and fine.

Is it because of my C-section that the baby turns out to be perfectly well, with no heart defect at all? Once again, she is returned to us. This time, we don't want to send her back to the nursery where the babies sleep, because we know the doctors will find something else wrong with her, and this time we'll never get her back.

~

Once I can stand at the window, holding my baby, the view is surprisingly beautiful. I hadn't known the hospital complex was this close to the water. In the middle of winter, the East River shines with silver light on Roosevelt Island with its bordered streets and clean squares of grass. The whole wall is clear glass; the view is a movie screen, a panorama. When I feel the worst and the loneliest and the most scared during the five days I'm in the hospital, I can watch it, reminded as I always am in New York, of the world outside myself, outside my body.

All I want is to escape my body that seems to have failed my baby daughter again and again. I can't walk, can't do more than a shuffle, I can't eat solid food yet, I can't lower myself into a chair to nurse my baby.

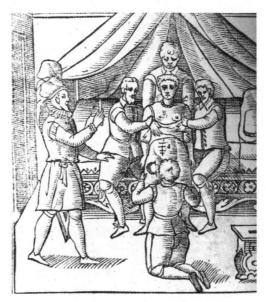

Four male assistants prepare a woman for a caesarean section; the physician stands to the left holding a razor. Woodcut by Girolamo Mercurio, 1651.

After the pregnancy, after the birth, I will forget warnings, medical tests, surgery, my hands tied down, incisions.

I will try to believe in this maxim because it is so often offered: *Focus on the baby.*

Because I love the baby so much. I adore her, can't remember my life before she was born.

But when I learn other women's birth stories, online, in books, in person, I'm the bad fairy in the story, sulking in the corner at the christening of a beautiful baby, thinking bad thoughts, thinking only of myself.

For years, I can't stand to hear anyone's happy birth story, and if someone starts talking about natural childbirth I can't help myself—I have to quickly leave the room.

~

Three years later, at a different hospital, I do it again. I give birth to a second daughter via C-section.

The story is all a tangle. If my C-section was so awful, why do I choose to have one again? If my C-section was so awful, why do I not blame the medical community? And why, if I could revisit my first daughter's birth, would I choose the C-section again if it would save her life? Do I know what I have missed by not having a "normal" birth?

Most of all: Why is the first person I blame always myself? For the difficult pregnancy, for the difficult birth, for the difficult days after?

Years later, as the mother of two daughters who I get to watch grown up, my sense of the experience is all contradiction. My daughters are beautiful and healthy. I am so lucky.

I don't want to lose this experience, have it fade from memory, but at the same time I also don't want to feel its rough edges anymore, always with me, a stone I turn over and over, concealed in my hand.

The late Polish poet Czesław Miłosz observed: "When it hurts we return/to the banks of certain rivers."

~

In the fairy tale, the mother never gets her daughter back. The mother's body is a country the girl departs from, forever.

~

An operation that virtually always resulted in a dead woman and dead fetus now almost always results in a living mother and baby—a transformation as significant to the women and families involved as to the medical profession.

⌒

The self did not unravel.

    The lesson was chalked on the sidewalk like a lost body, these lines the surgeon sketches—to save her, cut here and here and here—

reclaiming home birth and discovering HELLP syndrome

∿ *Daniela Montoya-Barthelemy* ∾

THERE WAS A TIME, up until about a year before I attempted my first home birth, when I would have easily opted for a C-section. The impression I had about birth was that it was dangerous and unpredictable. I thought our bodies were not to be trusted and were safest in a hospital with doctors to rescue us. Growing up Xicana in a small New Mexican town, I learned that if you could afford the hospital and formula you were not only better off, but you and your baby would also be healthier.

Though my career began in early childhood development, I strayed into social work and research. On my path toward a master's in public health, I avoided the child and maternal health track, wanting to prove that I didn't have to do *travajo de mujeres*. Even though I always knew I wanted children, I had no academic or historical knowledge about birthing. Nor did I have family experience, as my lineage no longer shared the birth room as a way of educating the next generation. In fact, I didn't know many pregnancy or birth stories from my family because they were regarded as private matters. I remember it was deemed scandalous and inappropriate when one of my eldest cousins sent my grand-parents some photos in which she was clothed except for her large pregnant belly. Our view of the body was through the Catholic lens of original sin.

As a physician, my partner Andre knew more than I did about birth, and had significant questions about the reproductive health system in this country. When he and I started talking seriously about pregnancy, we began reading about the history of obstet-rics, midwifery, and gynecology. Our discoveries floored me. With just a few books, research papers, and documentaries, my world was turned upside down. I learned my body was more than capa-ble of giving birth to a healthy baby. I found compelling evidence that births with the least interventions and interruptions are best for both the birthing person and the baby. I learned that the cae-sarean is a major surgery, often over-utilized in this country.

I also discovered how pregnancy and the birth process were violently colonized, institutionalized, and white-washed, under-mining women's and all wombholders' trust in themselves and their traditions. This process was part of the widespread loss of culture among indigenous women and women of color, and explained how I could be so ignorant of my own Latinx family's traditions in the birth room. In fact, it was when I joined white women's circles, looking for something I couldn't name, that I first encountered pieces of these traditions. The rituals and philoso-phies had been heavily reinterpreted and commodified but none-theless were born of the communities that bore me. I had uncovered fragments of my heritage and was ravenous for more.

I got pregnant while we were diving into our research. We began interviewing *parteras* and doulas in our new city. We had moved to Minneapolis, Minnesota for Andre's surgical residency program about a year before and hadn't yet found community. Some people back in New Mexico were supportive of homebirth but most of our family thought we were crazy. I didn't care. Enthralled by the wondrous abilities of wombholders, I readied one of the rooms in our new home exclusively for the birth, complete with yoga mats, a tub, and an *altar*. Andre and I attended classes in which we were the only brown people and the only ones planning a home birth. I felt empowered to heal some of the trauma that had filtered through those who had given birth in my family for generations.

At thirty-seven weeks and two days pregnant, I had an appointment with my midwife, Kate, and my chiropractor on the same day. An odd pain in my right shoulder had begun the night before. My chiropractor adjusted my back and the pain lessened. I mentioned my shoulder in passing to Kate, but neither of us paid it much attention. When the shoulder pain hadn't subsided after three more days, I was frustrated but far from alarmed. That evening, I told my husband I was planning an acupuncture visit the next morning. He agreed this was a good idea but thought we should check in with my midwife as well. It was after 9 PM, and I really didn't want to bother her. I was trying to be tough, but for hours my intuition had been telling me to call. Andre studied my face and body language and said he wanted to know for sure that it was nothing. After my text, Kate called us almost immediately. She asked some questions and sounded relieved at my answers. Just in case, she asked us to go get my blood pressure checked at the drug store and call her with the numbers. I grumbled about the cold but went. I was sure it would come back healthy and normal as always. It didn't. My systolic pressure was 160, elevated well above the normal range. Kate was unwavering; we had to meet her at the hospital. I burst into uncontrollable tears. I had no idea what could come next. But I gathered myself and asked if we should stop at home for an overnight bag. She said yes, but to be quick and throw in the baby's stuff just in case. I packed some clothes, toiletries, my makeup, and one random onesie. I was in complete denial that we would be coming home with a newborn.

Walking into the hospital beside Andre and Kate, I appeared calm and collected, but inside, I was shaking. I knew something was seriously wrong, and I wanted an out. We walked through those hospital doors and into the care of a doctor who Kate transferred to, when necessary. A nurse hooked my baby up to the fetal monitor and we were able to see that he was not in distress. They took my urine and blood, and Kate transferred my prenatal history. We learned there was some protein in my urine, but depending on another couple of tests, it didn't necessarily indicate anything dangerous. I would likely be sent home or kept overnight for observation, though there was a small chance I would need to be induced. As I looked around at the cold walls and busy strangers in the room, a pang of grief hit me. I mourned the calm and loving environment that our *casita* would have provided.

Our doctor brought in my blood tests and told us we could go home that night because everything looked fine. Andre, Kate, and I shared a deep sigh of relief. But before I could finish my next thought, a new team burst in the room along with a doctor who introduced herself as an OB/GYN. Apparently, the tests had been read incorrectly. In fact, my liver, kidneys, and blood showed an extremely rare disease called HELLP Syndrome: hemolysis (H), elevated liver enzymes (EL) and low platelet count (LP). Rather than going home, I needed to stay for an emergency caesarean. The room spun, and as I turned around to seek comfort, my doula appeared. I hugged her and looked desperately at my husband, who knew I needed more details and began asking questions.

The doctor explained that my liver enzymes were dangerously high, indicating that my liver was overworking itself. It would only be a matter of time before it, or my placenta, ruptured. It was my liver that had been sending pain up to my right shoulder for the last few days. Simultaneously, my blood platelets had dropped dangerously low, which could lead to a plethora of potentially fatal complications. This meant that an epidural was impossible, as I would be at a high risk for bleeding into my spine. I had to be put under general anesthesia.

There were so many people in the room, and it was all moving so fast. I sat there frozen, but all I wanted to do was run—down the hall, out the door, back to safety. My doula saw the panic in my face and asked if I'd like a minute alone to talk things over with my husband. I knew that line. I recognized from my own doula training that she was creating space for me to breathe. I gratefully said yes, I would like a moment. She moved to leave so everyone else would follow suit. Before they did, the doctors reminded me that I really didn't have much time and that the operating room would be ready soon.

I turned to my *quierido*, and even though I already knew what I had to do, I still asked, "Are you sure there's no way around this?" He explained that the placenta material was leaking through the walls of my uterus and my body was reacting to it as foreign. My body was basically attacking itself. He said that all of the research papers and case studies he'd found online in the last few minutes were saying that the only cure for HELLP syndrome this severe in a pregnant person is to get the baby out as fast as possible. I asked if he would help me make sure that they followed our after-birth plan for the baby, and he promised he would.

I spent the next few minutes trying desperately to get my dad to answer the phone. It was about 2:30 AM and he, along with most of my friends and family, lived more than 1,000 miles away. He was the one other person in the world I wanted to say goodbye to, and according to the doctors, we needed to prepare for the worst. When he didn't pick up, I called my sister. As I told her what was happening, she reminded me that she had preeclampsia with her twins and that the C-section was going to be easier and safer for me than the way I wanted to do it.

Her words took me aback. They embodied the colonized view of bodies and birth pervading our daily lives. I knew she was trying to reassure me that I was going to be all right. But she had planned her C-section before a slow onset of preeclampsia, while I was in a potentially fatal situation and without community, in the middle of the hardest night of my life. Nothing about this was easy or safe for me or my family. When I said goodbye, I felt even more alone. It was time to go into surgery.

Andre and I held hands as we made our way down the hall to the operating room. I said a few last words about our baby name choices and my wishes in case I didn't make it. Before the doors, we stood with tears in our eyes. I gave him one last steady kiss and marched into the operating room to climb up onto the cold table under the bright lights. No matter my fears, my baby deserved a chance and I had every reason to believe this was the only way to give that to him.

As they readied their instruments, the medical professionals made random conversation. The assistant anesthesiologist sat at my head and stretched my arms into a T. A nurse walked in, and without a word, uncrossed and spread my legs, which were covered only by the thin hospital gown. I immediately pulled them back together and lifted my head. She explained that she needed to catheterize me, reopened my legs even wider and pulled my gown halfway up my pregnant belly, leaving my *concha* completely exposed to the room of strangers as she inserted the hard tube into my urethra. The conversations and preparations continued. I stared at my reflection in the plastic light fixture and tried to tune into my strength and my baby.

The doctors moved closer to the table as they took a timeout to call out each of their roles in my surgery: "31-year-old female, operating room XYZ, caesarean section for HELLP Syndrome, OR nurse," etc. The anesthesiologist began to cover my mouth, but before he could, I remember saying something to the effect of, "Wait. I need to say something." I lifted my head and addressed the room. "Thank you each for being here in the middle of this night. Thank you for coming to take care of me and my baby. Please, please take good care of me and my baby. Thank you." They all stared at me blankly. I wanted to make them connect with us, to acknowledge the human lives they held in their hands. As someone bringing a new life into the world, I deserved that. As humans working in the sacred process of birth, they needed it. With condescending eyes, my surgeon looked at me and asked, "Okay, are you ready now?" Without waiting for an answer, she nodded at the anesthesiologist behind me. I placed my head on the bed and counted backwards as instructed. I prayed for my baby, connected to my husband's spirit, and dug into my strength.

The first time I remember being fully awake, I was being pushed down the hall to the room where my partner stood skin-to-skin with our baby boy covered in a blanket against his chest. As Andre handed me our *hito*, tears of joy and heartbreak streamed down my face, and putting my nose to his head, I breathed in his *olor dulce*. I recognized the movements of his tiny hands from what I felt in my *matriz* in recent weeks. Looking into his deep dark eyes, I realized I had known and loved him all of my life.

At the same time, I was awash with anger and grief. Something kept telling me this was not my baby. I stared at him, thinking, "How sad that you had to die." I knew it made no sense. But my baby, the baby I was expecting to push out of my body and pull up onto my chest had not yet been born and never would be. He had died.

The next fifteen hours passed in a painful but blissed-out blur of breastfeeding, fitful sleep, medical checks, and hospital food. I was so grateful to be alive and consumed with the care of my newborn, I didn't care how sore my *matriz* felt every time I moved. And I had no idea what was still to come or how hard recovery would be.

I would get more sick before I was well enough to be released from the hospital. I would be separated from my baby and placed in the ICU until my body slowly provided evidence that it was recovering. I would be returned to my room where I would have to fight to breastfeed my baby while being alternately supported and intimidated by multiple health professionals, all with differing opinions. I would get snide and racist comments surrounding our original plan to home birth from nurses who were caring for my *hito* and me in the most vulnerable states of recovery imaginable.

One nurse had introduced herself as a friend of my midwife, so I shared some details about our planned home birth and how devastating the emergency caesarean had been. Despite my situation, I told her I was still so enthralled with traditional medicine that I was considering a change of career to bring home birth back to more in the Latinx community. Her response was that it was a wonderful option for some but shouldn't be open to certain populations. She said our high health risks were giving home birth a bad reputation. I stared at her in disbelief as she walked out the door. Slapping me in the face wouldn't have hurt as much.

During the last conversation with my surgeon before we left the hospital, I asked why I had gotten HELLP and what I could have done to prevent it. She said if she knew the answer she'd be a millionaire. According to the research, there aren't any known genetic or behavioral risk factors for this life-threatening illness that occurs in less than 1 percent of births. She wasn't worried about it happening with me again because the recurrence rate is low. But she used this opportunity to warn me away from trusting my body, as I now had an "unproven uterus," weakened by the caesarean.

But the thing is, it was my body that saved me and my baby. By truly listening to my body's warnings, Kate, Andre, and I were able to work as a team to get the care that was needed.

At home, we had a couple of disjointed weeks together before my husband had to return to his surgical residency, working more than sixty hours a week. I had no idea what it was going to take to heal from this birth. No one had prepared me for the post-partum period of typical birth, much less a traumatic one. My scar was tight and painful when it came into contact with any-thing: a waistband, a countertop, a baby carrier. I peed con-stantly as if I was still pregnant and I didn't know why. And the core of me, my whole center, felt weak and disconnected, as though they had removed much more than just the baby during surgery. I was unaware of the underlying medical issues I was having, and my doctor thought nothing of these symptoms at my six-week follow up.

Most people I reached out to didn't understand why I was still holding grief when both my baby and I were safe. No one under-stood that I felt blessed and cursed. I was on a long, dark, lonely road to recovery, in a new city where we still didn't know many people. Most days it was just my *hito* and I, slowly finding our way. At first, I couldn't do much more than lie on the couch with him watching Netflix. Just making sure we both got fed felt like it took all of my energy. But eventually we developed a routine and grad-ually built on it. We'd get up in the wee hours every morning to nurse and see his daddy off to work. He came running with me, enjoying the view from his stroller as I attempted to quell my anxiety and depression. I even started the seeds of a new repro-ductive health business during his daily naps. And eighteen months of successful breastfeeding played a major role in saving our relationship and repairing my mental, emotional, spiritual, and physical health. It was the salve that both our hearts needed.

Our traumatic birth and my residual emotional and physical health issues have sent me on a quest to heal myself without a map or guide. On my journey, I've connected with teachers and learning opportunities in traditional womb health, holistic sexuality, postpartum medicine, and somatic psychology. It didn't take long to realize that this was more than a personal mission. I have fallen in love with the birth world, both intellectually and professionally. Reproductive health is the intersection of public health, social justice, and sexual health that I've always been searching for.

My son was six months old when Panquetzani, also known as Indigemama, traveled from California to present her workshop, Matriz y Concha, to the *mujeres* of the Twin Cities. For two days she led us through traditional practices for womb and vaginal health. She taught us why it's so important to work on the caesarean scar. And as she guided us in self womb massage, she strummed her *guitarra* and sang *La Llorona* while I touched my scar for the first time. I heard the whispers of my abuela's sayings, grounded in Panquetzani's ancestral teachings. As a *curandera's* granddaughter she holds sacred knowledge that has long been lost to so many of us. In this space, I met radical students, artists, mothers, doulas, midwives, and other reproductive health workers, some of whom were queer and all of whom were of color and/or of indigenous descent. I was home. This was the core community my heart had been searching for.

seam

~ *Cameron Dezen Hammon* ~

THE FIRST TIME I saw my mother's scar I was small and playing with her hairbrush. I was seated at her pink-tiled vanity, dipping my fingers in her creams and lotions, spraying perfume into the humid air as she stepped naked from the shower. The ragged line ran from her groin to just under her ribs, and looked like it had been drawn with a red crayon, like the seam on my Raggedy Ann doll. I lowered my eyes, embarrassed, and focused on her chipping toenail polish as she wrapped in a towel.

Before I was born my mother was a beauty queen and a beatnik. A Catholic, she was crowned Miss Pennsylvania Junior Miss and then became a civil rights activist, helping to organize campus marches in Pittsburgh and Ohio. I wanted to be like my mother in so many ways. I was like her in the ways I didn't want to be, but not in the ways I *did*. I become so still in anger that I frighten even myself (like her). I lack the extraordinary focus she's always had—either with a cause, or a career (unlike her). And physically, our bodies are opposite; though petite, she is broad shouldered and long-legged. I am small everywhere, unremarkably built.

My grandmother's body was nothing like my mother's body: She was tall and elegant, and, I learned recently, gave birth vaginally. I'd always believed my grandmother had had a C-section like the rest of us. I assumed she shared our seam, which, from that first sighting in my mother's bathroom had become, for me, a symbol of what we survive, of how we endure.

My grandmother was a single mother. Her husband had a second wife and family in the next state over and upon discovering this, she left him. Her parish shunned her though she fared well on her own, working as a secretary at Melpar, a Cold War government contractor. There she met a brilliant, depressed, nuclear scientist, whom she later married. He gave them all a new surname, *Loving*, and he was. But things got hard. He attempted suicide one summer night by rigging himself to the basement generator in their Cape May home, while my mother and father ate dinner upstairs in the kitchen. My grandmother survived all this, thrived, even, though my understanding of my grandmother's strength has always been tied, in my mind, to her C-section. As it turns out, something else held her together. What, exactly, remains a mystery to me. She has been dead for thirty years, but if she were alive I would ask about her labor. Were her slender hips just wide enough to let a baby pass safely? Was her pelvis a degree to the right or left of where mine sits?

When my mother had me in 1975 she was thirty (or thirty-one, or thirty-two; to this day, she won't tell me her true age), and they were ripping vertical seams in birthing women. When I was pregnant in 2006, she told me the story of my birth: the cry of *infant distress* rising up like smoke in her hospital room, of being wheeled into the OR and then seeing past the privacy curtain, of watching the doctor's reflection in the polished chrome cabinets as he cut her from sternum to pubis, then pulled me, blue as a stone, from her womb.

Though my father didn't want children, my mother told me he paced the hallway outside her operating room, nervously handing out cigars. She said he called all of his friends, shouting, "It's a girl!" It was a rare joy between them. In the end, my mother survived my father. She held it all, and us, together.

My OB induced me on a Thursday at my last office appointment, a few days before my due date. She said that my fluid was almost gone, that my daughter couldn't stay inside me without it, and I wouldn't be leaving the hospital that day without her. Though I was tired of being pregnant, I thought the decision to induce had something to do with my doctor's weekend plans. I'd been gorging myself on Internet paranoia and had begun to see my kind doctor as the *medical establishment* bent on thwarting my well-researched *birth plan*. And besides, my brother's rock and roll band was performing a concert in Brooklyn that night, and my mother would most certainly be there. Couldn't this wait? I could have a baby without my mother, I thought, but did I want to? I called her from my Houston hospital room, panting between contractions. She balanced a Cabernet in one hand and her phone in the other. "Cameron's in labor!" she shouted at the crowd, and passed me to one, and then another of my New York friends. I heard a cheer go up. I passed the phone to my husband, and then set about sweet-talking the anesthesiologist for more Demerol.

After twelve hours of a Pitocin drip, and waves of stabbing contractions, I pulled my knees back in the angled hospital bed and pushed. *No C-section*, I murmured, mostly to myself. I pushed for three hours. Later, I thought I must have looked like one of those Samurai figurines, in the squat before the kill-lunge.

Three hours is too long to push, and the fetal heart rate monitor chimed. As mine had in my mother's uterus, my daughter's heart rate dipped, and dipped again, every time I contracted. Suddenly, my noisy hospital room became very quiet. The nurses moved in synchronous action. With a few snaps and tugs, my bed slid away from the monitors and into the hall toward the OR. I jabbered to the nurses in a drug-numbed patois, inhaled their perfume, complimented their eyes, their hair, as they silently wheeled me into surgery.

I couldn't see past the privacy curtain. There was silence after the sawing and grabbing was finished. Not the squall I had expected. Could they botch this? It seemed improbable. But there was a moment, maybe just a second, in which I didn't care if they did. I was tired. So tired. And then I heard it, the holler. Like a woman in a well.

"She pinked up quick," my doctor said, and handed her, mewing, to my husband.

A few weeks later, I was in my doctor's office for a follow-up exam. "I wouldn't have known from looking at you," she said, "but the birth canal is tilted." She was hidden behind the sheet draped across my lap, my feet freezing in the stirrups. "There are some things you can only see in surgery," she said, and later, in her office, added what was perhaps obvious: My daughter would have never made it out without a C-section. Three years later, when I struggled to get pregnant again, my doctor explained that the tilted canal is a genetic abnormality. "It's a trait that mostly died out," she explained, "because usually mother and daughter carrying it died in childbirth." The genetic blueprint of our twin affliction would have died out, too. But this trait reappeared, or we who carry it did, after the proliferation of C-sections.

My scar is what my fertility doctor calls "slash and go." "Sometimes you only have a minute," he says gravely. Though it saved my life, and my daughter's life, I suspect that my C-section—or rather the scar tissue that resulted from the emergency, "slash and go" nature of the surgery—may have made my womb an inhospitable place for a second pregnancy. But I can't be sure. Though I have been pregnant only once in the eight years since having my daughter, a pregnancy that ended in miscarriage, I can't bring myself to have the other surgery that would tell me for certain. My husband and I are mostly resigned to being the parents of one. But as I approach forty, almost a decade since I had my daughter, I wonder what another child of ours would be like. Would we have a son? Or another daughter? One born, perhaps, with this same tilted pelvis that I have? Yet, I don't make the appointment. I don't schedule the surgery. Instead, I finger the still-numb parts of my scar. I touch the ragged seam that runs the width of my body like a boulevard, and wonder what it holds together in me. I trace its length and slope and imagine what my daughter's will look like.

the parent room

∿ *Rachel Moritz* ∾

FOR EIGHT DAYS AFTER my son's birth, I lived in a room off the neonatal intensive care unit (NICU). I was the only parent staying in this suite of four rooms—each with a single bed, a couch, and small fridge. There was just enough space at the foot of my bed for Finn's bassinette, and after he was unhooked from IV antibiotics, he spent his days with me. At night, I delivered him to the nurses and crashed in shifts interrupted by the phone's strident ring. "He's hungry," a nurse announced when I picked up the receiver. Then I shuffled down the hallway to the NICU, a room that blinked with alarm lights and swirling computer screens. The preemies slept motionless inside their incubators, pacifiers looming against their tiny faces. Finn, in my arms, looked giant by comparison, long and lean in the baby blanket brought from home. After we nursed, I swaddled happy monkeys and balloons around him and returned to my Percocet sleep.

We both slept better in those first nights apart. During Finn's entire babyhood, he never rested well near me, not in the side-sleeper we tried for a week before I hauled it to the garage, nor in bed, held tightly against my chest. I often wondered if our early separation had marked him. The first time we tried—night

five of our NICU stay—my partner Juliet was there to sleep on the
pull-out couch. No one rested. Finn's face puckered in fury, his
crying relentless through the long hours. At 4 AM, the staff changed
shift, and a nurse we hadn't met before, young and buoyant in her
white sneakers and smock, knocked on our door. She took one look
at Finn and announced that he was starving.

"Don't be so proud," she said. "You need to ask us for help."

This nurse disappeared to the front room and returned with a
formula dispenser and plastic nipple cover. While Finn drank
deeply, she doled out suggestions meant only to be helpful. I
needed to follow a strict two-hour feeding schedule, she said,
pinching Finn's cheeks as his eyelids fluttered shut. I should pump
to increase my milk flow and supplement with formula. Most
importantly, I should be open to learning anything and everything from the nurses.

How to say this: Though she helped feed my child that morning, I hated her advice. Living in the NICU was like living in a
zoo, a circus ring. Everyone watched you, rightfully assuming
ignorance. There were lessons and admonishments: Don't even
consider co-sleeping; What do you mean, you don't want him to
have a pacifier? Sucking is a natural instinct for babies. Or, whispered in my ear late at night: Don't you want to cover yourself
up while you nurse? I was so tired I let the hospital gown fall to
my waist; the nurses insisted on pulling a screen around my chair.

And there was something else beyond this public existence difficult for an introvert. The NICU staff assumed we were a family.
They assumed Juliet was Finn's second parent, already on the
road to legal adoption. They assumed Finn was my first child,
which meant there would be a second. They assumed no interior-
ity, which also meant no doubt. What they assumed was that I was
a mother: a machine of a person doing, feeding, caring. Their
watchful eyes meant there was no going back. It was my job to

keep this baby alive. And perhaps that was the biggest shock of all. He was *my* baby.

~

Finn's conception: Our doctor pedaled over on her city bike, a catheter wrapped in the bag pulled from her basket. She was taking a break between the main course and dessert at a friend's, her cheeks flushed with wine. Eileen was my GP, a former home-birth midwife who worked at our clinic. She had offered to help with my inseminations, free of charge, in the comfort of our home—a great gift. And here we were, Juliet holding a flashlight at the foot of our bed, Eileen unsealing the vial of sperm from donor 4XXX, a twenty-something industrial designer who described himself as a lover of mountain biking, sculpture, and his family. A willing-to-be-known donor whom my child could contact when they turned eighteen. I had selected him in a rush when our first choice at the sperm bank—a quiet minister who loved his LGBTQ friends—was suddenly unavailable. With this donor, I'd gotten pregnant on my third try, miscarried seven weeks later. And now, the shipment paid for, Eileen on board for the narrow window of ovulation, I could choose someone else or cancel the month's attempt.

Did my rushing mirror something of the chaos of creation—relying on instinct, giving up head control? As if there was any-thing instinctual about it. Juliet was out of town when I called in my order. We argued on the phone. She felt rushed and wanted to study the online database more carefully. I wasn't sure if she was right, but chose 4XXX nonetheless, possessed by a mixture of urgency and doubt I couldn't shake in the days following.

Because, if I'm honest, my journey toward Finn was consumed by ambivalence. There had never been a time when I didn't want a child—but, oh, the complications. I fell in love with Juliet when

I was thirty and married to a man who wanted to have kids, with me. Leaving the marriage was momentous, a step toward some greater happiness that I desired with every part of myself. I just didn't want this happiness to be childless.

Standing in Juliet's kitchen months after we met, I hooked my thumbs through the belt loops of her jeans and asked, "Don't you want to have a baby?" "No," came her clear reply. I couldn't accept this answer. I held a vision, a literal picture in my mind, which had materialized during one of our phone calls, my legs stretched against the wall and Juliet's voice in my ear. I saw us standing in a field together, in summertime. A tall boy leaned against me, the top of his head almost reaching my chest—he was maybe eight or nine. This boy felt real but was gone in a flash.

Our relationship continued, as did my question of choice. Was a child essential? It felt like standing on a bridge across a perilous canyon. On one side, there was something I wanted—time to write, think, and claim space for my life—but in that plunge, too, there was terrible grief. On the other was the child my body and heart wanted, but also, fear. I was scared of my sister's life with two boys under the age of five—their constant activity, the exhaustion I felt after only a few hours at their house. And there was the risk of raising my child alone, of Juliet leaving.

I understand these anxieties now, from the other side of parenthood, as the concerns of a younger person unable to deal with loss. I wanted a baby but feared the undeniable changes it would bring. The mindfulness of queer parenting, all the planning required, would have stretched me in the best of circumstances. Under the strain of different desires, Juliet and I were pushed to the brink. We did couples counseling with three different therapists. We set up a trust that would make my sister guardian if anything happened to me. We even bought a small duplex so Juliet could live upstairs, myself and the baby below. We'd see how it went, we told friends. I would parent the child and Juliet would be auntie. And then, when we were finally ready, had chosen the sperm bank and donor, begun the monthly ritual—the flashlight, the catheter, the small vial warmed in my palm—when I was in fact already pregnant but didn't know, Juliet's father died by suicide. Finn's conception was round two, after a miscarriage and pause in the darkest of times. I was thirty-six years old and felt I couldn't wait any longer.

After Eileen pedaled off into the night, Juliet washed our dinner dishes while I rested in bed. It was like this with our inseminations: a tense aftermath in which we each took space. A candle flickered on my birth altar, beside the bowl of water poured that morning, the infant cap I had found in a curbside free box. My baby was a spell I would summon with these charms, asking the spirit to come to me. Conception was many things—mental, spiritual, psychic. Physical was the only thing it wasn't.

During those four days of labor, we didn't know the baby was a "he," just a process working its way through my body, pushing against my cervix, which didn't open and didn't open—never beyond three centimeters—for hours before the C-section. What I felt about the process included a large dose of anxiety; how was the baby mine?

Was I too scared of the pain to "raise the intensity," as the head midwife advised when she visited my room on Tuesday night? I'd been laboring since Sunday, at home the first twenty-four hours, and in the hospital another day and night with little progress. My contractions were four minutes apart, as they'd been all day. The midwife took my hand and looked directly into my eyes. Did she know she was telling a woman who'd been racing laps for hours that she was only walking, or at best, lightly jogging? I was certain there was no way I could birth this baby. But I mustered my strength, asking for a few moments alone. Juliet left the room. In my maternity sweatshirt and hospital underpants made of coarse beige gauze, I sat on the bed and told the baby I was ready to meet them, I wanted them, and everything would be okay. Instantly, a rush of liquid trickled down my leg as the next contraction gripped me.

After Finn's birth, replaying the sequence of events in my head, I realized this was my water beginning to break, a slow leak that continued through the night. Because I didn't know to tell anyone, the midwives kept up their cervical checks, and by the time Finn was delivered on Wednesday afternoon, an infection in my placenta had spread to his lungs. Maybe I could have prevented this.

Tuesday night, I followed the midwife's advice, trying to raise the intensity of labor. I circled the hallway, gripped the railing when contractions took hold. We tried more squats and standing, the warm pulse of the showerhead, Juliet and our doula pressing my hips. Later, I would learn that my entire labor was prodromal, never clicking into active rhythm, though the pain and exhaustion was real. Hours passed. By midnight, I only wanted sleep. I asked for the epidural.

~

The skin touch of Finn when I finally held him. My ankles were swollen, club-like on the wheelchair foot rests. My body was a drugstore: Percocet and Motrin for pain, surgical anesthesia, morphine from a few days earlier when the midwives thought my contractions would strengthen if I slept through the night.

I didn't recognize this baby inside the NICU isolette. He lay on his back, one hand taped to an IV port, a fluff of blondish hair on his well-shaped head. Of course, I remember thinking: It hadn't been pushed through my vaginal wall. The nurse helped position him on my chest, and he drank a little colostrum. I stroked his cheek, watched the pulse of his throat as he sucked. It was hard to leave after only an hour.

No one woke me that night, and later, even today, I wondered why not. Did a nurse rock Finn when he cried? Did they feed him formula? The next morning, I woke filled with despair. When I managed to sling my legs over the side of the bed and stand, leaning against Juliet, I wept with exhaustion and pain from my incision. After nine long months of pregnancy and four days of labor, was this feeling all there was? I sobbed until the top of my hospital gown was soaked. Then the phone rang. It was a nurse saying, "Your baby is hungry," as if this were normal news. And mother that I was, there was no time to cry. Again we wheeled down the hallway. Finn was wailing, and this time we fumbled as he latched on and slipped off, the morning nurse hovering with suggestions on technique.

~

A persistent regret in those early days; I never saw our placenta and umbilical cord, two features of my pregnant body that felt like ghost children themselves. They had been packaged up and sent to a medical closet deep in the bowels of the hospital. I asked one of the midwives if there was any way to find them. Could I take the placenta home to freeze? She said it wasn't possible; they were stashed somewhere as evidence. It was all unclear. Of course, this was nothing compared to the difficulties of Finn's birth: the emergency C-section after his heartbeat started dropping, the infection that filled his lungs with fluid. He was whisked away to the NICU for a mandated ten days of antibiotics. I couldn't hold him until late that night, when the distracted nurse in charge of my post-op finally wheeled me down the hall.

The larger challenges of my passage into motherhood: I didn't find a known donor in the way I hoped, and didn't have a partner giddy or excited about my pregnancy. Our birthing classes; Juliet and I awkward in the rows of straight couples who inhabited a space they never had to question. I went alone to hospital tours, to my midwife appointments, to my ultrasounds.

I'm struck by how much of Finn's birth story still resonates with loss. The losses I encountered while trying to bring someone new into the world, which was ultimately a gain. How some losses continue; they're part of the story. Like Finn's paternal line, which I sometimes imagine as a dissolving wall in a room that continues expanding.

But when I share my sadness with other parents—in the moments when we tell our birthing stories—I'm immediately washed in self-loathing. What luck, I hear the voice inside me say, to deliver a healthy baby. Why call his birth difficult when it was basically a privilege? Why waste time envying another woman's eight-hour labor, her easy sleeper, her second baby? So what if our family's formation was messy, if we weathered a storm to emerge intact on the other side? The C-section, after all, was not without a silver lining. Juliet was the first to bond with Finn, following him to the NICU while the surgeon sewed me up. Her palm warm on his belly; she kept watch. "He's really, really nice," she said when she came back to sit with me. Given her devotion to Finn today, her singular role as co-parent and beloved playmate, it doesn't sound like much. But I knew in that moment she was smitten.

⁓

While pregnant, I imagined my child as the Sun card in Tarot: an exuberant naked boy riding a horse. The bringer of joy. The card

smiled from my birth altar, came with me to the hospital where I
propped it against the rails of my bed. It spoke of collaboration
with the universe, a mystery I couldn't understand. My child made
of science and luck: the bulky tank filled with liquid nitrogen and
propped in my car's backseat. I had picked up my order at the
FedEx station, stood in line with strangers who watched me carry
it to the parking lot. Driving home, I eyed the tank through the
rearview mirror. I thought how strange it was that a single vial
inside connected me to someone I didn't know.

And often when I felt my baby's hiccups or the drift of a heel
across my belly, I was seized by this undeniable fact: I didn't know
the donor. Only his boyhood photograph mailed by the sperm
bank, along with his one-page interview and health questionnaire.
This boy, at three or four, sits on the steps of his childhood home,
dressed in blue overalls. He holds a stick in one hand, and he's
serious, staring straight at the camera. I didn't know him or his
parents taking the photo. My God, I would think, the breath catching inside me, what on earth had I done? These people were strangers, and my baby was a stranger, too. Inside my belly he slept and
kicked, especially late at night. His essence felt peaceful, as if none
of the anxiety riddling my mind had anything to do with him.
Though during his birth, we faltered together and couldn't make
it work. In the parent room that housed us afterward, I was not
fully his mother but inching my way there.

Today, I remember the room in still life, as if no other mothers
have stayed there since, risen by the phone's ring to tend their
newborns. The mauve walls, with their strip of floral wallpaper,
are lit by the battery-powered candles I bought for labor and never
used. On the bedside table, there are flowers from friends, a book
I still believe I will read. My nursing pillow is propped on the
couch. My slippers wait by the door. But Finn and I aren't there
anymore. We've moved past this room into the flow of his

childhood, which is a space I can only describe as fully embodied. His pleasurable heft in my arms when I carry him, his face pressed against mine.

So here's another take on his birth, one that turns from loss. In the minutes before the C-section, Finn's heartbeat dropped dangerously, and the midwives raced my gurney down the hall. It was a dreamlike panic, as if rushing to a death. I focused on my breathing: steady, steady. I closed my eyes, the haze of fluorescent lights against my eyelids. I wanted to keep my baby alive. And mercifully, once the OR doors swung open, his heartbeat steadied. The midwife held my hand. Juliet's eyes, nose, mouth—everything else covered in a white cap and gown—appeared by my side. I was crying when they pulled him out. She stood to peer over the drape. "It's a boy," she said, without affect or surprise. Then the boy's clear cry, the strangeness of his cry because it sounded like a baby you would hear in a film, carried by another woman. But this baby, this boy, was mine. We waited. The nurse brought him beside me, his long fingers curled to his face. I stroked his cheek and said, *Hello*, and my voice calmed him instantly; this baby knew me. He stopped crying before the nurse carried him away.

PART THREE

Beyond Postpartum

Aroutine C-section is a brief, major surgery involving a four-to-six-inch incision in the uterus before removing the baby (or babies), umbilical cord, and placenta. The surgical team then sews up the uterus and closes the abdominal incision.

This is a tidy description. The recovery is typically described in simple terms, as well. A C-section is viewed as comparable to other abdominal surgeries. Post-surgery, mothers are advised to follow instructions that alleviate serious complications (e.g., a wound opening, blood clots, infection) or after-effects deemed normal (e.g., abdominal pain, weakness, persistent bleeding). It can take six weeks or longer for mothers to feel strong and well enough to lift a baby, walk, or take up their usual activities. While C-section mothers are advised to be cautious and attentive to their bodies, it's striking that much of this mirrors advice for vaginal birth.

Standard instructions tend to deemphasize the high rate of postpartum complications and the missed opportunities in preventing these complications. NPR and *ProPublica*'s 2017 article, "Nearly Dying in Childbirth: Why Preventable Complications Are Growing in the U.S.," points to the ways U.S. culture tends to marginalize postnatal experiences, mainly focusing on the health of the mother only while she is pregnant.[1] As a result, after nine months of careful attention and concern, many postpartum mothers are left to wonder if what they are experiencing, physically and psychologically, is acceptable or usual. Sometimes they don't take their pain seriously enough; sometimes, it's too late.

The physical body is not always in step with procedures and recommendations. Just as we experience differences in our physical healing, our psychological healing, which facilitates our physical well-being, varies. Those of us who have given birth by caesarean may be offered prescriptive advice about our postnatal bodies, but even conventional discussions about the after-effects of caesareans end at the arbitrary six-week cut-off described for all births.

Across this collection, individual agency is an important topic that connects to the scarcity of conversations concerning caesarean bodies. The essayists consider what agency means across many roles: as mothers, parents, patients, providers, and more. These considerations link intimately to how our ways of giving birth reflect cultural values, technologies, power structures, and market forces. Birth is highly personal *and* shaped by circumstances — racism and sexism, identity factors such as class, hospital policies, medical decisions, geography, access to support and wealth, and much more that can fuel our unique reactions to pregnancy, labor, postpartum, and beyond.

The essays in Part Three go beyond postpartum, resisting conventional explanations for varied scars. They unveil social and cultural disparities that can intensify these scars. They offer portraits of overturned expectations and questions when bodies diverge from plans. They tread themes connected to grief, death, depression, social judgment, silence, and resistance. They seek understandings beyond acceptance or closure and remind us of the ongoing need for transparency, care, and birthing justice. These essays speak to how our ways of giving birth thread deeply into our psyches.

birth and death and what gets cut away

~ *Catherine Newman* ~

I'M THINKING OF BIRTH, even though this is not birth. Or it is
the birth of death, though we don't understand this yet. Also,
we do understand. Both things. Where I'm sitting is on the floor
outside the bathroom where my oldest friend—my dearest of
forty years—is struggling. She is home from the hospital; she
has been *debulked*. They've butchered out as much of her ovarian
cancer, and the neighboring afflicted organs, as is surgically
feasible and humanly endurable. Her colon has been sected and
resected. Resection, C-section. I am full of advice. The similar-
ities are not irrelevant, but they are terrible. "After I had Ben,"
I keep hearing myself say from outside the doorway, cringing.
Life and death, and the constipation is the same.

After having two kids, I know this: In the Venn diagram,
"C-section" overlaps with "debulking" at *constipation* and *infected
sutures*. "Scheduled C-section" and "emergency C-section" over-
lap at *constipation, infected sutures*, and *baby*. One circle is otherwise
filled with smiley faces; the other with Edvard Munch's *The Scream*.
Ben's sister Birdy's birth was a choreographed waltz of nurses and
instruments: a temperate, predictable sequence of cutting,

stitching, and getting born. Ben's was more like a strobe-lit horror-movie rave, the kind that goes blurry and death-defying after someone slips you a roofie. Were the twenty-six hours of labor surreal? They were. Blood, blood, and more blood—"Is this too much blood?" a nurse asked our midwife, who shrugged in an unsettling beats-me kind of way—and also pain, the kind of pain that makes you think in slappingly fresh clichés, as if you're inventing them on the spot: like a jackhammer, like a monster, like a bed of nails, like a ring of fire that actually catches your spinal cord on fire, too, so the whole thing is up in flames, lava pooling in your bowels, erupting in your brain stem, so not a ring of fire as much as the 1974 movie *The Towering Inferno*, Steve McQueen ideally on his way to rescue me from the blazing passenger elevator. I said one thing, one time, that entire day of my life, and it was, "Kill me." The baby was a deep abstraction, swimming safe somewhere beneath the circling sharks.

But it *was* too much blood after all! It was a placental abruption, and this sequence of things happened: My partner Michael and our friend Sam split a Snicker's bar, passing the candy over me like I was more picnic table than flaming supernova; they discussed the proper seasoning of vegetarian curry; I dilated seven centimeters and then no more; the anesthesiologist arrived to offer me the blessing of an epidural; they "lost" the baby's heartbeat; an alarm went off; people surrounded the bed; someone yelled to me to get on my hands and knees and push; I got on my hands and knees and pushed. "How did you do that?" Michael asked later. "Weren't you technically paralyzed from the waist down?" This part of the story feels apocryphal now, but I swear I hoisted myself onto my hands and knees and pushed, like the mother lifting a Volkswagen overhead to rescue her child.

And then they were wheeling me into the OR, and Michael was holding my hand, but his teeth were chattering, and everything telescoped: the baby. The baby. All those stupid printed onesies and little socks and plush rattles, the changing pad Velcro-ed so optimistically to our dresser. The icing on the cake, but there's no cake. Garnishes, garnishes, parsley, lemon wedges, and nothing's on the plate. A body with no heart. Just proliferated objects of loss, meaningless limbs and organs. We were going to go home with empty arms. They were swabbing my belly yellow, scissoring off my shirt, and we were going to go home with empty arms. "Please!" I said, and Michael kissed me—they were making him wait outside. "Please!" Empty arms. I could feel the crushing weightlessness of it. We were going to have onesies and socks and rattles and no baby. It was shockingly chaotic, the machines, people yelling for this and that, the anesthesia, waiting for the anesthesia to kick in. "Don't wait!" I said, crazy. "I don't care if it hurts! Just get the baby!" (Note: They do actually wait.)

Then a dull slicing, a dull tugging, pressure, pressure, pressure that's the same as pain but without any edges, and then a vast slippery sliding. Aloft! A giant purple baby! A giant purple, then red, then pink baby, all squinched up like an enormous angry frog, its face bisected by a comically huge, tight-lipped frown that opened into an enormous hole of yelling! The baby! The baby! I drowned in relief, died from it, lived again, and was temporarily paralyzed and ill from relief and medication, for hours on end, while friends and family partied with the baby in the other room. My kids thought I was kidding about this, but it's true: In the video recording, colorfully dressed people dandle Ben and kiss him, pass him around like a shared trophy, while—look close and you can actually see this—in the background I am as swaddled in bandages as a mummy, barfing quietly into a bowl.

"Are you disappointed not to have had a vaginal birth?" people asked me, for weeks, months, years to come, and it always made me laugh. Like asking the rescued if they were sorry to have left their monogrammed luggage aboard the *Titanic*. I didn't care! I didn't. Except that the post-surgical grossness blurred a little into the trauma. "Watch your stitches!" a nurse yelled through the closed bathroom door. "Let it come without bearing down."

"I don't think a whole lot's going to happen without bearing down," I yelled back. "This thing's not about to slide out on its own." That thing had as much in common with poop as concrete has with a milkshake. These were the days of stool softeners and glycerin suppositories, of constipation becoming a strangely persistent subplot in the story of my new life as a mother.

And meanwhile, in a parallel subplot, I had gone crazy. Technically, I think this was PTSD, but there was nothing *post* about it. The trauma was all-consuming and ongoing: I couldn't live without the baby; I had almost lost the baby; I could lose the baby. "You're going to need to get a finger up in there, loosen it *digitally*," the nurse said through the bathroom door, as matter-of-fact as a drive-through attendant. *Burger. Large Coke. Stick a finger in your own asshole*. Okay. Torn vagina or sliced abdomen, incontinence or bikini scars. These were not my issues. This new ancient face, these rosy lips, swallowing, swallowing, breathing, asleep. My issue was adapting to the heartbreak of human life. My issue was learning to love through the potential of unendurable loss. Some part of me had been sected away with the baby. Something was gone. I had been debulked.

Years later, in the email in which he'd announced his wife's pregnancy, a friend of mine wrote—with self-conscious humbleness —"We just hope that everything is fine." As if that's such a modest wish! When really it is everything. I laughed, but not in a good way; more in the mentally ill way of a person who ducks and yells, "Choppers incoming!" every time someone makes a smoothie in the blender.

And I am thinking of this again, on the floor outside my friend's bathroom. We are laughing and crying. We have not talked about poop this much since we were six. She has a headache so dully crushing that she is sitting on the toilet with an icepack pressed to her forehead. "I can't," she says, because, despite my running to the pharmacy every few hours, despite the prune shakes and the stool softeners and the glycerin suppositories, I am now offering the nurse's final, terrible piece of advice. The *finger* advice. My friend is laughing and laughing now. "I can't," she says. And she can't.

Did I recover? Maybe. I don't know. It's better than it was, when we got the first roll of film back from the processing lab, and it was me and the new baby in our rocking chair, and, just outside, framed in our bedroom window, the menacing face of our clinically deranged neighbor, peering in. We had no idea. Danger was everywhere, seen and unseen. The beast, the shadow of the beast, the beast's scat, steaming in the sun. How do you love when there's loss, always looming? How do I now? And I don't know the half of it. In three years, in the middle of a terrible night, the hospice nurse will unhook all of my friend's tubes and wires and bags and drips of output and input—"Just this once. Just for a few hours." We will pull a clean, dry nightgown over her head, and she will crawl into bed with me. I will hold her in my arms, her body like a milkweed pod that's gone to fluff, her teeth huge inside her smile that's shining at me in the dark. I'll be thinking (and I'll be wrong again) that this is as hard as it gets. Love in peril. Loving a heart that could stop beating. Loving with your own stretched and scarred organ, the one that might pound on long after, like a dumb animal. Like it didn't get the memo about what the heart can take.

the zig zag mother

⁓ *LaToya Jordan* ⁓

ON A STAGE IN a hushed theater, a magician escorts his beautiful assistant to a vertical box with three doors. He helps her in, then shuts and locks it. The assistant's head and hands are visible from holes in the front of the box. She is trapped, but she smiles, knowing the audience is in for a treat. The magician sticks two blades in the box, one at the chest and one at the belly, separating the box and beautiful assistant into three sections. She smiles and waves as he pushes the middle box out to the side. It looks like her midsection has been cut out, leaving her body in a zig zag, a square-shaped hole where her belly should've been.

This is how I choose to see the birth of my daughter. I'm a Zig Zag Mother. As a writer, I try to spin my trauma into beautiful scenes. Symbols help me cope. It's the way I sort out my feelings.

My daughter was born on a sunny spring day in 2012. I had spent my entire pregnancy preparing for her arrival, watching documentaries about birth, doing prenatal yoga, learning hypnosis for a more relaxing delivery, taking a class for parents birthing at home or in birth centers, readying my mind for her entrance into this world through my body. Wanting a natural or unmedicated childbirth contrasted with what I wanted when I was eighteen and told my mother, "No baby is ever coming out of my vagina!"

My fascination with childbirth began when I watched the PBS Nova episode, *The Miracle of Life*, with friends. I was a teenager, and it was my first time seeing a baby being born. I was fascinated, but horrified. Back then it seemed scary and inhuman to push a baby out of my vagina. I tried to get my closest friends to promise they'd act as my surrogates in the future.

Pregnant at thirty-three, I watched hours of YouTube births, mostly unmedicated and usually water births at home and in hospitals. I watched a few women receive epidurals. I'd watch them on mute so that my husband wouldn't think I was losing it—he thought I was spending too much time online reading about childbirth. I cried every single time a mother held her new baby, covered in goop, to her chest. I'd pause the video on that moment, the look of joy on their faces something I desperately wanted to experience. I also prepared myself for the possibility of an epidural, reading how important it was to remain still as the needle went in your back. I watched a few C-section births, but it wasn't my plan; I wasn't going to be *that* woman. Surgical births seemed sterile, devoid of the raw animalism of vaginal births. And my husband and I spoke about not having a C-section as if it were something we could control. I wish I had watched more of these blue-curtained births.

Here's how I thought my daughter's birth would go: Contractions would start, and I'd walk around the apartment, occasionally stopping to get the lower back massages my husband had learned from our doula. We'd call our doula and the midwife on call at our birth center. Our doula would meet us there. She and my husband would help me through contractions. I'd feel the need to push, and we'd sit in the bathtub. I'd push and push, growling like a lioness. I'd feel my daughter's head crowning, her shoulders would come out, and then I'd pick her up out of the water, my blood and cheese-coated baby, and everyone in the room would

be crying. I didn't expect it to be magical. I knew it would be
tiring and hurt like hell, but I still thought it would be the happiest
day of my life.

My water broke around 2 AM. When I got to the birth center,
two midwives examined the amniotic fluid leaking into my
Depends diaper and told me I'd probably have to transfer to the
hospital. It was the color of split-pea soup, indicating there was
meconium in the amniotic sac. It could've coated her lungs and
blocked her from taking her first breath. I labored at the birth
center for nine hours before transferring to the hospital in a bumpy
and painful cab ride. I still thought I'd get to have a vaginal birth,
with or without an epidural. I labored in a small triage room with
my husband and doula supporting me, hooked up to a machine
that monitored the baby's heart rate. The day moved slowly until
suddenly there was a rush. My daughter's heart rate was slowing
with each contraction. After an additional seven hours, I still
hadn't dilated. I was given Pitocin to speed up my labor, and an
epidural for the pain and in preparation for a possible C-section.

The obstetrician on call performed a final cervical check to
see if I was progressing. After she took her gloved fingers out of
my body, she looked up at my face and shook her head back and
forth, her blonde ponytail dancing behind her head. She told me
she was sorry. I asked why.

"How did you get that scar?" she said, pointing to my face. The
room buzzed around us.

"Car accident," I said.

"I'm sorry. You're going to have a C-section and the incision
will probably end up healing like the one on your face. Was it
hypertrophic or keloid?" She shook her head again, as if I were
her child and had a skinned knee.

The scar on my face is smooth, wide and stretched, no longer
bearing the signature bubbly and raised look of keloids because

steroid injections flattened it. I didn't care how a scar I'd be able to hide would look. I was worried about my baby's plummeting heart rate, and, although I wasn't in pain—because of the epidural, I was tired, scared, and ready for this to be over.

"But you can definitely VBAC," the doctor said. In one of the books I read about the high rate of C-sections, a VBAC was the dream of every mother who had an unwanted C-section. The chance to do it the "right" way the next time. Later, I would cling to that information.

On the operating table, I wasn't prepared for the pain of a C-section. I thought I wouldn't feel a thing. The doctors kept saying, "It's pressure, it's pressure," but I assured them it wasn't. I kept saying, "It's burning, it's burning." I don't know what exactly I was feeling, maybe the scalpel cutting into me on my left side? I smelled what I assumed was my singed flesh. The anesthesiologist increased the medication and then everything was numb, not just my body; all the emotions sucked out of me, too. I was disoriented. I knew I was there for the birth of my daughter, but I was also confused about why I was there and what was happening to me.

While they cut through layers of my skin and delivered my daughter from my body, the medical team talked about what they'd order for dinner: Chinese or pizza? I don't remember what they agreed on while I was having a profound, life-changing moment. Then there was the yanking. The baby was lodged near my hip. I wondered if this was what being disemboweled felt like. I felt full. Then I felt nothing.

After a while—it could've been fifteen minutes, a half hour, or hours—I heard a baby cry. It took seventeen hours of laboring, first in a birth center and then at the hospital, for my daughter to be born, at 7:22 PM. My husband was joyous: "That's my baby. That's our girl!" I looked at him, standing behind my head. I was embarrassed that he was making such a scene. He saw our daughter first, held her first. But I, the person who protected and carried her for nine months, was supposed to hold her first. He placed her head near my head. I said, "Hi, baby." Seeing her was the only time I felt something good in that operating room. I couldn't reach out to touch her, but my husband put her cheek against mine. She was bundled up like a burrito, her eyes coated in goo, but after she heard my voice, she turned her head in search of me, like she was being reunited with an old friend. Her seeking face pierced through the haze of anesthesia. She knew me, and that is the moment I hold onto.

The day after giving birth, I saw other mothers walking the halls, standing upright, while I circled the floor bent over like I'd just been punched. I couldn't stand up straight because of the pain. I left the hospital walking like someone with severe scoliosis. On the first night we were home, our daughter woke up in the early morning crying, and I shot up out of bed, forgetting about the four-inch incision and staples holding me together. Two sections of my skin were in a painful tug of war. I couldn't get out of bed, even to get my kid. It was the first time I felt like a failure as a mom.

During my first few weeks as a mother, breastfeeding was difficult and exhausting. My daughter didn't know how to properly latch, so every time I tried to feed her it hurt, and we were both frustrated. We were supplementing nursing with formula. I thought I'd already failed her and risked her health by having her cut from my body. (She didn't get all the good bacteria from my vagina that could, I had read, prevent her from having asthma, allergies, or becoming obese.) I became determined to do whatever it took to make breastfeeding work. I couldn't also give her formula when *everyone* knew breastmilk was best. I would not let my body fail again. We hired a lactation consultant, and my doula also came over to help. I spent hours online, in forums, and sitting on the couch trying to make it work. By the time she was a month old, we finally had gotten the hang of breastfeeding.

But I was still angry, at myself and everyone else. We had taken a natural birth class, and I started to get emails with class members' birth stories. Reading about their successful water and home birth stories made me jealous. In class, I had judged those families for not choosing safer births. What if something happened at home and they didn't have time to transfer to a hospital? But I started to think I should have planned a home birth. Three other couples planned deliveries at the same birth center we used, and all of them transferred to the hospital as well, with one other mother having a C-section. I was furious with my birth center and my midwives because I felt that they misled us about the hospital transfer rate. I was furious with myself for switching from an OB to midwives. I loved my OB, but those water birth moms in the videos were the ones who looked the most ecstatic, and I had wanted that for myself. If I had stayed with my OB, maybe I would've had a vaginal birth.

As I searched for symbols for the womb, I learned that Pandora's box was not a box, but a jar large enough to fit an adult body. My uterus had become my Pandora's box. With each stroke of the scalpel, deep fears, emotions, and doubts escaped my uterus. I wanted to shove them all back in. What had I done wrong? I had midwives, a doula, a birth plan. I read all the right books. I had practiced self-advocacy. I knew to say no to Pitocin. I thought I was prepared.

I blamed myself for being too crunchy, too modern, for wanting to experience the searing pain of vaginal birth. I wished I had never watched Ricki Lake's *The Business of Being Born*. I should've just gone with my OB to the hospital and had an epidural. I found a way to blame my C-section for everything and anything that didn't go according to plan: motherhood, breastfeeding, diaper rash, sleep problems, low iron, and not being able to stay home full-time.

I saw a therapist. We only had two sessions, but it felt good to talk to someone about how I was struggling and second-guessing every decision I made. How could I trust myself to make good decisions moving forward? Should I quit my job and stay home with my baby? Was I even in the right career? Should we move to a different city? Besides my precious daughter, was there any beauty to be found in my birth experience?

I desperately wanted to know what led to my C-section, and my therapist encouraged me to find out. At my six-week appointment, my midwife said it started with the meconium, and then the baby had moved into a sideways position and wasn't budging, that her oxygen was being cut off and her heart rate dropping with every contraction, that she had been at risk for cerebral palsy. But I didn't believe her. I believed the perspective that my C-section was inevitable because I had 1) gone to a hospital, 2) was hooked up to machines and not allowed to walk, 3) had Pitocin, 4) had an epidural, and 5) hadn't dilated fast enough for medical staff. I had joined and reinforced the statistic that more and more women were having C-sections because hospitals were trying to get babies out as soon as possible. I found out that the hospital I transferred to has the highest birth rate in New York, that I had been placed on the conveyor belt in the baby delivery factory.

When I told people about my trauma, they usually responded with, "At least you have a healthy baby!" It shut down the conversation about my birth experience and left me feeling guilty. And what about the mothers who had lost babies? They'd trade places with me in a heartbeat. So, I shut up about it.

Being a Zig Zag mother means my plans have changed. I left the operating room a different person. To get to my uterus, doctors pushed my intestines and bladder out of the way, and I don't think I was put back correctly. I was rearranged as a mother, as a person. My husband and I had always thought we'd have two children and planned to space them two years apart. But when my daughter turned one, I wasn't ready to start trying. Year after year passed. I kept telling my husband I might be ready soon but that having another child would be the biggest "taking one for the team" ever. I'd joke and say I'd have another kid, "only if I can never work again" or "only if you buy me a house." When my daughter turned four, she started asking for a little sister. At check-ups, my gynecologist would ask if I was planning to have more children. I'd say I was on the fence.

One thing that kicked me off the fence: another surgery. In 2016, I had a fibroid inside my uterus surgically removed. The fibroid had been causing heavy, painful, and long periods, and the blood loss made me severely anemic. I asked my doctor if she could guarantee that I could VBAC after the procedure, but she couldn't.

In surgery, where my doctor used a tool to remove the fibroid in pieces through my vagina, she discovered it was bigger than she had thought: seven centimeters, the size of a tangerine. She switched to a laparoscopic procedure to get the rest. That second uterine surgery took future vaginal birth off the table. After the procedure, my doctor warned me not to wait too long to get pregnant because fibroids commonly recur and, at thirty-eight, my window of fertility was rapidly closing. She said we could start trying as early as three months post-surgery.

That three-month time frame terrified me. Putting a deadline on the process made me less ready and more fearful of having another child. Under no circumstances did I want another C-section, but I wanted another baby and didn't have a lot of time. Three months passed. Another year of seesawing. Forty loomed, and I knew it was time to decide.

It seemed like every time I thought I might be ready to take one for the team, a story would pop up in the news of a woman just like me: Black, in her thirties or forties, who died after childbirth, usually post C-section. I consumed article after article about Black women dying at higher rates in childbirth: *ProPublica*: "Nothing Protects Black Women From Dying in Pregnancy and Childbirth;" *The New York Times*: "Why America's Black Mothers and Babies Are in a Life-or-Death Crisis;" *CNN*: "Childbirth is killing black women in the US, and here's why." One day I spent hours reading about how Judge Glenda Hatchett lost her daughter-in-law to internal bleeding after a C-section. And then there was the story of Shalon Irving, who had a fibroid history like mine and died of high blood pressure a few weeks after she gave birth to her first child.

While I had read plenty about birth complications prior to giving birth, I hadn't seen anything about how my race was a risk factor. Now the stories of Black mothers dying were everywhere I turned. I saw my face in those photos. It didn't matter how many books I read or videos I watched, how much prenatal yoga I did, or that I had health insurance, college degrees, a steady job, and a husband—none of that had saved any of the Black women I was reading about.

In 2018, Serena Williams went public with her scary complications after her C-section: blood clots in her lungs and internal bleeding. Had she not advocated for herself multiple times, requesting specific tests because of her history with pulmonary embolisms, she might not be here, either. If someone like Serena Williams still experienced doctors discounting her pain and symptoms, why would medical staff listen to me? I had a good medical team during my pregnancy, but the anesthesiologist hadn't believed me when I said I felt burning pain during surgery. It was only at my husband's insistence that the anesthesiologist increased my anesthesia. It's hard to advocate for yourself when you are sick or in pain and there are white coats and green scrubs telling you they know best. I also had plenty of experience over the years with doctors who didn't treat my pain seriously—such as when my former doctor told me to take ibuprofen after I told her my periods felt like I was being stabbed with a hot poker. Judgments were made about me based on preconceived notions about Black women. I liked my original OB, but I thought it was weird he kept referring to my husband as my boyfriend and I wondered if he did the same with his white patients.

To me these statistics and inequities and memories are life and death possibilities. I have a wonderful child. If I had another C-section, I could die from a blood clot traveling to my lungs; I could bleed to death; or I could have a stroke or a heart attack.

So I asked myself if I was willing to put my body through the wringer again. Was bringing another life into this world *that* important to me that I would risk my own health and life? Was I willing to die for an imagined human being when I already had a family?

The answer is a resounding *No*.

But it's not an easy no. I'm now forty and my fertility is waning. Every month when my period arrives, I think how my chance at having another child fades with each drop of blood. And I realize that my eighteen-year-old self was right: "No baby is ever coming out of my vagina!" It seems a weird thing to mourn, to miss a vaginal childbirth. But I'm also mourning the fact of not having another child born of my body. It's such a final statement, one that makes my heart long to travel back in time and change the past. There will always be a part of me that wants to feel life growing inside me again. That hunger hit watching my friends at forty experience their firstborns, and I have a feeling the ache will be greater when I'm menopausal. But there's another part of me that is growing stronger the more I say, I don't want to be pregnant again, that I don't want another C-section. This is a reclamation of my body. Being pregnant, delivering a baby, breastfeeding, and recovering from major surgery were all experiences where I felt like an alien in my own body, where I wasn't in control. I get to say no more, not again. But this is not a "no" to a second child, just a no to my body as a means to an end.

On days I'm feeling like that out-of-whack Zig Zag Girl, not the person or mother I thought I'd be at this age, I comfort myself with the fact that there are different ways to become a mother. I am lucky to have felt what it is like to grow a human, but ultimately, it's my desire to mother that I want to fulfill. My husband and I have discussed the possibility of adoption to expand our family and spent months going through the process to become foster parents. We recently welcomed a baby boy to our family for as long as he and his family need us to care for him. When I'm holding him close, smelling his baby smells and listening to his sweet sighs, my heart says mother; it doesn't matter that he wasn't born of my body.

It's been six years since my C-section, an experience that left its mark in more than one way, the most physical being the scar that almost no one sees except for my husband and me. That moment changed the trajectory of my mothering. And, though I'm still trying to get past the fear and trauma, they've also forced me to look at new paths, new ways of being. Sometimes, when I'm feeling down about not birthing another child, I touch the scar. It is tough, smooth, but thick. It's a line in the sand now, a line I don't want to cross again—but it's also proof that I was the mother who was cut in half, and I lived to tell the tale.

CBAC

～ *Judy Batalion* ～

"DON'T MOVE," my anesthesiologist barked. "This is the most critical moment of the entire procedure!" He turned to address his team of scrubbed-in minions. "If this goes wrong, her spine will be ruined. Forever! Plus— no baby."

I was hunched over in the middle of the arctic OR. As if I hadn't had enough trouble with airflow in my pregnant state, the enormous fetus pressing on every organ, now my neck was bent down, compressing what was left of my pathway. *Breathe*, I told myself, as I'd told myself a few hours earlier, when Dr. Crazy waltzed into my pre-op area. "There are three kinds of epidurals we can give you," he had explained. "What would you like?"

What would *I* like? Was this a restaurant? You're the world-class specialist, I hadn't said.

A high-risk case, I'd been to the hospital over thirty times in this pregnancy, and no one had once mentioned that, at the last second, I'd have to select the paralyzing drug for my second C-Section. The nurse, who'd been prodding my arm with needles as if it were the plastic film covering a microwave meal, had rolled her eyes. "I'm extremely anxious and have trouble handling injections," I'd said. "I'd like valium."

I'd been serious, but Dr. Crazy laughed. I'd told my husband
to run down the hall and ask my OB what drug I should select,
while Crazy quizzed me about my Jewish roots and how I'd come
to New York from Montreal, then presented a tirade about the
challenges he faced in anti-Semitic Russian medical school and
his son's woes in current training.

"I don't feel good." My words were tinny in the cold metal
landscape.

The OB residents asked me questions to calm me down, keep
me aware.

"Don't talk!" Dr. Crazy screamed. "Pass me the vial. No, the
other vial! Watch me. The whole birth depends on this moment."

"I'm really not feeling well," I said, as Crazy circled an area
on my lower back, a patch I almost never saw and could not picture. I managed to move my hand over my stomach and pet myself
calm. I grazed my scar, the same scar that had been ripped open
three times ("put in Velcro!" my OB once joked), the vertical mark
that cut through me like a permanent *linea nigra*, splitting my sides.
I thought of my skin, how it was not just a boundary but composed
of layers, filled with tissues, dimensions of soft organelles. I tried
to remind myself that I could breathe within its thickness. "I can't
breathe. I'm fainting."

They laid me down under a bouquet of spotlights. "Give her
oxygen."

"You all right?" Dr. Crazy asked.

I nodded.

"Now I have to start all over again." He sighed. "Don't worry;
I like a challenge." I was lifted back up. Again, my back, motions,
wipes. Nameless people came in and out; machines wheeled by.
I looked down at my old friend the hump, memorizing its shape.
My baby. I was about to meet my little girl.

This is why people "go natural," I thought. This is why they have doulas who they've met more than two minutes before. Give birth in warm water, in their Brooklyn galley kitchens with their husbands, best friends, and husband's best friends cheering them on by their sides. This is why they take the pain. Now my arms were being spread out, held at my sides, and I couldn't reach my tummy, couldn't hold her, and oh god.

~

Abdominal surgery had saved my life. When I was a teenager, I suffered from acute ulcerative colitis (UC) and spent the better part of my twelfth to fifteenth years cramped in pain and hemorrhaging in the hospital. My colon was disintegrating like a shedding snake, refractory to an increasingly long list of medications. When all that was left was experimental drug trials, I insisted on removing the whole organ. I underwent a new procedure in which my large intestine was amputated and my small one reconstructed. Two surgeries later, I went from life in the bathroom to the café, from a morphine pump with proctologists to wine coolers with kids my age. I was cured, liberated, elated.

Eighteen years later, I stared at two parallel lines on a stick, shocked that Jon and I had conceived so quickly. My colorectal surgeon emailed me saying, "do NOT have natural child birth," and, "you MUST have a C-section," and I didn't question it. I also didn't mind. I knew that women who'd had my UC surgery had low fertility rates, and I felt tremendously lucky. Natural birth risked ruptures, incontinence, and further gastric surgeries. I didn't want to ruin the sutures that had kept me together for so many years. But, more than all that, I could not bear the idea of prolonged labor, of amorphous abdominal aching. The resulting agony of surgery, I knew, was pungent but contained, tied to the physical slice, which felt more manageable.

I did not think physical prowess (which struck me as the epit-
ome of patriarchal standards) would make a difference to the
quality of my mothering. My own mother was an anxious depres-
sive, a hoarder with paranoid tendencies, so the fact that I emerged
from her naturally didn't make much of a difference. I had spent
over three decades trying to clean up the psychological and
domestic mess around me. I became an academic art historian,
worked in white-walled galleries, explained creativity, looked for
answers. My own home had white sofas and almost no other furniture. My mantra was "less is too much." I was drawn to straight
lines, sleek geometry, schedules, plans in advance.

Wanting a C-section was not, to say the least, a popular stance
in my bohemian, feminist, intellectual milieu. I understood my
friends' and colleagues' skepticism. I had studied medicine as a
cultural and political paradigm. I spent a summer working for a
Breast Cancer Action group, teaching young women to take
charge of their own mammary health. I had written a dissertation
about feminist art and psychoanalysis. I was not naïve to "the
man." Yet the surgery I had experienced as a teenager had never
felt like something done to me; rather, it was a process that had
allowed me to take control over my body.

The pro-caesarean taboo was so strong—even more so than
feeding a baby formula or a toddler juice—that I stayed silent
about my slant. When my prenatal yoga teacher learned I had to
have a C-section, she called out, "remember to refuse the Demerol!"
I said, "OK," but thought: I needed Demerol just thinking about
it. When the uber-trendy lactation consultant asked why I had to
have a C-section, and I explained "due to serious surgical history"
(when really I wanted to joke "to maintain the integrity of my
lady parts"), and she said, "I guess that's fine," I bit my
hormonally-swollen tongue. "I can find you a good OB who would

do natural," a friend's doula offered, and I replied, "thanks," knowing I'd never follow up.

When people judged my birth mode, like they judged my consumption of tiramisu (fetal alcohol syndrome!), Diet Coke (addiction!), or even bending down to tie my shoelace (suffocation! Your vagina will fall out!), I let it be. When everyone around me was talking about "taking back birth," I did not say, "I trust medicine," did not say, "didn't you have four rounds of IVF," certainly did not say, "I don't want it back." Instead, I spent my days seeking more surgeons, trying to find the most revered colorectal specialist who had OR time at the exact same time as my high-risk OB in case there were complications. While others were eating spicy foods to get things going, I spent my time clutching that baby in, praying my body would not go into labor before the set surgery date.

The night before my first C-section, my all-male planned-labor team, consisting of my dad, brother, and Jon, took me out for pizza. I thought: *The next time I eat I'm going to be a mother.* Three hours later, I felt a snap. Then, a toilet bowl of blood. Carwash between my legs.

At Labor and Delivery, the doctors took their time. I wasn't dilated, but I was starting to contract. Jon and I improvised Lamaze. We panicked and laughed and took selfies of both of us in blue hairnets.

Then, I didn't feel well. Really not well. When I tried to explain to the nurse that my insides felt gummy, my mouth was swollen, and I couldn't talk, she banged on the monitor twice then pressed the blue button on the wall and suddenly I was pounced upon by a dozen doctors, beeping, pressing, pushing Jon out of the way. I was wheeled into the OR, and then—black.

An hour later, she was on me, warm, perfect. This thing that was of me and not me, weighing on me again, but in a different

place, a new way, a companion to the air, the light, others. My
body was confused. My limbs felt foreign; the baby, still me. *My
baby. My baby is alive.* She lunged for my breast before I had a
chance to panic about football versus sandwich holds.

"Imagine," I said to Jon, "if we'd had a water birth. A self-guided
guru delivery in a forest. In a five-story Victorian walk-up. Dead.
We'd all be dead."

When other moms pitied me for my horrific, 1950s patriarchal
experience, for not remembering the morning I gave life, I sighed.
But internally, I smiled. Once again, surgery saved me. And this
time, it saved my baby too.

～

I'd been told that eighteen months was physically the best time to
start trying for number two. I was now thirty-six years old, over
the advanced maternal age line, and, lo and behold, I felt a famil-
iar uterine tug.

But—the test was negative. Then my period started. And it
went on. And on. Several doctor visits later, another test indicated
that my HSG was rising. I *was* knocked up. Only, the unusual
period was not stopping either. *Some women bleed*, my OB said, but
the increasing amount was alarming. I did not feel well. I fainted.
I went to emergency. The OB began monitoring me every
forty-eight hours—for six weeks. It could be a miscarriage, an
embryo lodged in a vein, the death of a twin, or worse, ectopic.

The pregnancy seemed to be growing, but so were my symptoms. The embryo remained invisible in all invasive ultrasounds.
No one could find it, and it definitely was not in my uterus. My
hormone levels seemed unusually low, but my doctor put off any
action. A cousin who was a physician became anxious: Your tubes
could rupture. You could die. Your doctor doesn't want to be sued,

a friend told me. A wrong abortion is the most expensive mal-practice suit in New York State.

At ten weeks, I was back in emergency in the middle of the night with sharp shards of pain running inside my thigh. The neonatal radiologist said he thought he might see the embryo in the lateral edge of my right tube, but he wasn't sure. Finally, my OB called in a GYN to make the call. Take it out, *now*, it was decided: I would have to immediately be injected with a chemotherapy drug that would, hopefully, kill the fetus, growing like a destructive cancer in whatever organ it happened to be lodged inside.

"Why did this happen?" I managed to form the words, my mouth like a desert.

My OB shrugged. "It could be random—1.5 percent of preg-nancies are ectopic. Or, it could be due to your colitis surgeries. Scar tissue can make organs fuse, stretch or misalign. Internal adhesions can cause fallopian blockages."

Of course, this was the infertility risk I'd always heard about, but it made no sense. I'd become pregnant so quickly, twice. Plus, the OB who did my C-section two years earlier had noted that the uterus seemed clear. "Could it be," I asked, "scar tissue from my C-section?"

He paused. "Possible. Some new research is finding that link."

What had I done to my unborn baby, desperate to attach to me in the right ways but blocked?

Back home, I lay on my couch, feeling the wringing, the abortion at work, the fetus being absorbed into my own blood-stream, thinking about how we are not only our dead ancestors, but also our dead children. I didn't know what upset me more: that there was no explanation, or that the ways we heal come back to haunt us.

A week later, as my two-year-old Zelda sat on my lap while I read to her about Olivia the pig, the words stopped coming out. My lungs felt corseted. I pushed my daughter to the side, making room inside me, but no oxygen could enter. There I was, alone, with my toddler, about to pass out. By nighttime I was back in emergency. A possible pulmonary embolism. CAT scans, X-rays. But no. It was in my head, said another doctor. Just stress. (Just?) A week of intense Valium. Then another emergency: full-body hives, itching, burning, my skin on fire. Ice baths, hot compresses on my lungs. Severe allergies to the cat scan dye? The chemo? No one knew. More doctors. Emergency room. Steroids. Doctors. Waiting rooms. Months passed as I puffed on inhalers, feared smog, subways, Sundays.

Zelda must have noticed my anxiety, noticed I was afraid to be alone with her, that I was living in my head, trying not to think about how I'd never make life again, about surprise endings. "I don't love you, Mommy," she said as I tucked her in one night.

"What?" I knew I had to stay cool. I kissed her cheek.

"Too wet, Mama." She wiped it off. A phase? A silly phrase?

I took her small hand, clasped its softness in mine, dry from medication and weeks of staying inside. She slipped her hand out. "I only love Daddy."

For months, I'd been jealous of how Jon—whose mother had prioritized their domestic life—was the cook, the bather, the doer, while I—who'd never been taught to make toast, let alone dust— was the planner, the organizer. But now it hit me: skin to skin. Jon had done it; I'd missed it. Because of my C-section, I'd foregone the ultimate bonding experience, the template for all of Zelda's attachments. It was bad enough I was anxious, emotionally and physically absent over the past few months of illness, but I'd been absent at my only daughter's birth, unable to comfort her as she came into the world. I was like my mother, blocked from my daughter as she had been from me.

I thought of that birth day, the plummeting fetal heartbeat, the seconds of missing oxygen, and now the faulty implantation, off by just a few millimeters. It was all so fragile. The smallest things had the greatest impact. I'd been stupid to dismiss my friends. My C-section had ruined everything, damaged the foundation of my relationship with my daughter, and possibly every relationship she'd ever have. I was a fraud who hadn't really given birth. And now, I'd never get pregnant again. Medicine had deceived me.

"I'll tell you exactly what's wrong with you," said the pulmonologist Jon had talked me into seeing.

I'd been on the recovery warpath. Must heal, breathe, make children. Psychotherapists. Yogis. Physical therapists. Scar tissue massage. This pulmonologist, the best in the city, I was told, had sent me for my millionth round of lung function tests, touched my fingers, looked at my chest, and refused to listen to my version of my history. Yet he had a firm diagnosis.

"I feel like I can't breathe right now," I said.

"I know." He said. "I can see by how you're clutching the chair. Your problem is your brain. You have a faulty neural mechanism. Your lung function is perfect, but for some reason, your brain is telling your lungs that it doesn't take full breaths, when it does. Then you hyperventilate, and cause yourself to experience the very problem you fear. You can stop it. When you feel out of breath, just tell yourself what's going on."

Forty-eight hours later, oxygen poured through me. I felt like I was walking on helium soles. Thanks to the medicine man, I was re-awake, alive. By explaining myself to myself, I stopped choking. All I could control was that—my sensation. My perception.

Six months later, despite the tests that had revealed that my hormone cycles had never fully rebalanced, despite the X-rays that showed a fully damaged fallopian tube, despite doctors saying it would never happen naturally again, I saw two parallel lines. Flushed with estrogen and joy, I thought of how sometimes the things that made no sense turned out to be the best things of all.

This time, I found a C-section class at the uptown progressive birthing center. Taking back the C! I was ready to go with my flow, natural, gentle. My way.

Jon and I were the only people that showed up.

"I've already had a C-section," I explained to the maternity nurse. I felt confident, buoyant. I wanted to share my story.

"Why not do VBAC?" the nurse asked, excited.

"I can't," I said, but my voice wavered. Maybe I should have looked into VBAC, considered risks beyond ripping my own stitches, selfishly. I tried to touch my stomach but the maternity pants were pulled too high, and all I felt was polyester.

"Let's review the complications for future pregnancies," the nurse began. "C-sections can cause infertility and stillbirth. New studies show ectopic risk."

Yes! I wanted to clap. Finally, someone was warning me.

"The most important thing is not to let them take the baby away from you." Now my heart raced. I knew what was coming. "Even for a minute. You must do immediate skin to skin."

Over the past months, Zelda had been particularly loving, only occasionally recounting her preference for Jon. Perhaps her hostility toward me had been a phase. Perhaps I'd made more efforts at being present. I was starting to think it wasn't due to missed skin to skin, to that one moment. Her relationships with her parents were complex. A psychologist had told me her rejection of me was her way of testing boundaries, which she'd only do with someone she felt particularly stable with. The thing is, I'd never really know.

"They will try to take your baby away from you, even to another floor, to bathe her, to wash off the blood. You must never let them!" The nurse was on a roll. "You must insist on sleeping with her every night, on being with her at all times. During the operation, you will smell your own flesh being sawed apart. You will hear the saw. They might even take out your organs. This will give you horrific gas. You should make an eye blink code with your partner in case you are accidentally paralyzed."

Holy shit.

But, as she went on, it struck me that I'd had none of these problems the first time around. And what if I wanted them to take my baby to the nursery for a bit? What if I was ill, needed to heal, needed rest?

"Ask your OB if you can burn your favorite incense during the procedure. Tell them you want your music on the speakers, and let them know how many palpitations you'd like the umbilical cord to have before the cut."

I tried to imagine my OB, the House MD of high-risk maternal fetal specialists, doing surgery to Euro-trance and vanilla-scented candles as we group-counted peristalses. I'd come here eager for preparation, itching to share my story with other moms, wanting advice, tips, support. Instead I heard: the C-section is a sentence doomed to happen to you, and you will suffer afterwards, too. But I had already learned: sometimes it was all right to give in, to just breathe.

~

"They're at the uterus, about to take her out!" Dr. Crazy, the anesthesiologist, announced. He'd finally switched conversation topics from the glut of Albanians ice fishing in Quebec, which had kept him entertained until now. Once I'd been frozen (*do you feel this?* he had asked as he jabbed a wooden stick into my thigh), the screen between my face and stomach put up, and Jon was seated by my side, Dr. Crazy had become a friendly chatterbox. Who knew this guy, *this*, would be the backdrop to my birth? But as I caught Jon's rolling eyes, I was also grateful for the comic distraction to what was indeed the smell of and sounds of charring self, the hazy sensations of pressure and pulling.

My C-section was all medical, but after weeks of pre-labor contractions, I was so glad to be here, in one piece, awake, among surgical hands that I trusted. My CBAC, or see-back, I mused.

"She's out!" Excited voices across the room.

"Is she OK? Is my baby OK?"

She answered directly. A howl, the howl of my heart. They lifted her over the curtain—she was red, screaming, covered in black hair. Jon got up to cut the cord. I could not see, but I didn't count pulses. Then, they took her. Not far, just to one side of the room. "Go to her," I told Jon, and then I felt it—empty.

People sewing my stomach, doctors joking about lunch, cries cries cries. *Give me my baby!* I felt sick, I understood, I wanted that baby on me, in me, with me. Not because it was necessary for the baby, but for me.

At the end of forever, a wrapped, bathed baby was placed on my chest. I curled upward as far as I could and kissed her lips, thinking not of the slew of mistakes I'd make as I fumbled to pick and choose approaches and advice, nor of the wildly unpredictable trajectory of our love and lives, but feeling her warm velvet cheek firmly touching my own.

when expectations go up in flames

A Mother Rising from the Ashes

~ *Sara Bates* ~

IT STARTED TWO YEARS AGO on my bathroom floor. The pregnancy test next to the sink loomed above me, as I sat on the cool tile and watched the clock. Two minutes felt like an eternity when I was waiting to see if my life was about to change forever. The timer finally buzzed, relieving my agony. Two pink lines. My pulse quickened as I scrambled to hide the evidence beneath the sink. I was between the flannel sheets before my husband came upstairs to kiss me goodbye. He didn't suspect anything, even though I was sure my haywire heart bulging baboom-baboom through the comforter would give me away.

I wanted to take another test. I'd done my research; the first pee of the day could not be trusted. Still in bed, I downloaded *What to Expect When You're Expecting* to my Kindle. Later that evening, after I'd read a few chapters and peed on another stick, I told my husband the news. We were going to be parents. "Holy shit," he said, his eyes watery. *Holy shit.*

Those first chapters of *What to Expect* taught me I was already two weeks pregnant. With only thirty-eight weeks to learn every detail about pregnancy and motherhood, I quickly replaced the stack of fiction on my bedside table with books about pregnancy, baby gear, infant care and, in an effort to maintain my dignity, an occasional funny mommy memoir. Then one day I turned on my Kindle and discovered a new pregnancy genre dominating my recommended reading list: Natural Childbirth. *What to Expect* was still strolling through the produce section (*Your baby is the size of an avocado!*), so by that point in my pregnancy I'd invested more time locating my next Saltine than thinking about my child's birth. I took the bait.

My natural birth education started with *Posh Push: Modern Girls Reveal Secrets for a More Natural Birth*, filled with stories of women who'd delivered babies naturally after pregnancies filled with self-affirmation, yoga, and meditation. Alongside these beautiful birth stories were warnings of the risks associated with medical interventions during childbirth: spinal headaches, permanent nerve damage, vaginal tearing, difficulty breastfeeding and bonding with baby and, of course, the coup de grâce, unplanned caesarean birth.

Reciting birth affirmations sounded more pleasant than vaginal tearing, so when I finished *Posh*, I immediately Googled "how to meditate during pregnancy" and signed up for a prenatal yoga class. Then I devoured Ina May Gaskin and *Birthing from Within*, and hypnobirthing and *Hypnobabies*. I soaked in as much as I could, with the exception of information on caesarean birth. Those portions I skimmed. After all, I was taking such care to educate myself about natural birth and unnecessary medical interventions that I didn't need to study surgical birth. C-sections were for women who hadn't done their research or their yoga. I was healthy, strong, and prepared.

Each night before bed, I visualized my happy place, the sugary beach from my honeymoon in St. Lucia, where I planned to retreat during powerful "pressure waves" (because hypnomoms don't use the word "contraction"). I daydreamed about the moments immediately following my delivery, when I would hold my baby skin-to-skin before nursing for the first time. I interviewed a doula, but she'd been so distracted by her children during our telephone consult, I convinced myself my husband would be a more attentive coach, despite his reluctance to read hypnotic birthing scripts to me before bed or even finish his assigned reading.

In the days leading up to my due date, I bounced on my birthing ball and took long, warm baths, all the while reciting pregnancy affirmations. *I am a strong, capable woman. My body was* made *for childbirth. I* trust *my body to* know *how to birth my child. I* deserve *to have the birth I desire. I* will *have a peaceful, natural birth.*

Then, on October 9, 2013, at 1:38 AM, thirty-six hours after my water broke and three days past my due date, I was carved open like a jack-o'-lantern. A healthy, eight-and-a-half-pound baby boy with a sticky black traffic cone head was pulled from my belly. I'd been marked in the records as a case of "failure to progress" after three hours of fruitless pushing. Failure to progress was quite the mindfuck for a Type-A who'd devoted the past thirty weeks to controlled breathing, deep squats, organic coconut oil massage, and red raspberry leaf tea. Despite all my preparation, I failed to show up in the delivery room with my strong, capable body made for childbirth. Instead, I was an onlooker in a paper cap with tubes in her nose. *Pay no attention to that failure behind the blue curtain!*

Three weeks later I was back in my bathroom examining my deflated middle. The robust belly I'd nurtured for the better part of a year was an unrecognizable, doughy mass. I lifted two fistfuls of the skin that flapped over my pelvis to reveal the nearly toothless grin of surgical glue and tape stretching between my hip bones. My obstetrician had said the tape securing my incision would fall off within ten days; my husband had told me not to pick at it. I tried to decide which of them I wanted to strangle first as I scratched at the loose edge of a strip of tape then slowly peeled it off.

~

When I was pregnant no one told me about the silence of new motherhood, and it definitely wasn't covered in the recommended reading. A grandmother with the wrong shade of red smeared on her teeth once rubbed my belly while cautioning me about the sleepless nights and, oh, the crying! I'd been worried about the crying, and the musical toys and all the other noise, but it was the silence that did me in. After the visitors stopped coming and my husband arrived safely back at his desk and the baby finally closed his eyes, the silence would settle around me like a fog.

I spent hours holding my son as the combined weight of his body and the dense silence pinned me to the sofa. Then my postpartum persona, mad as a hatter from the sharp drop in hormones, would tiptoe into my head commanding my attention. *Why did you call the hospital when your water broke? You* knew *you should have waited!* After she tired of visiting me on the sofa, the hormonal bitch started to show up all over the place, day and night. I'd hear a deafening ring in my ears during my shower as I washed sleep and tears from my eyes. *It was a mistake to accept the epidural even though you were exhausted from hours of active labor. You should have held out longer. You were weak.* A relentless taunting rattled my brain at 3 AM, during my son's fourth feeding since sundown. *You shouldn't feel upset about your C-section; your son is safe and healthy. Why are you so selfish?* The sleepless nights, inconsolable crying and general uncertainty about absolutely everything related to caring for a tiny human were hard enough to manage without this toxic opponent in my head. Motherhood was kicking my ass.

When my self-doubt and regret weren't paralyzing enough, I'd top them off with a generous floater of paranoia. For extra kick. *Do you really think my water broke? What if the doctor lied about how fast I was dilating? Do you think the nurse fed him formula in the nursery?* My husband, whose distaste for my natural birth "hocus pocus" ran deep, just stared at me when I'd mustered up the courage to ask him these questions. He reminded me that our son was healthy and that it was time for me to just get over it. *All fair points, but try again, buddy.* He didn't realize how much I would have loved to get over it, how much I was struggling to dig myself out.

Forgiveness seemed like an okay place to start. I sent a fruit arrangement to the maternity wing at my hospital and, rather than writing what I'd really felt on the note—*thanks for the fucking C-section, ladies, and for making my nightmares a reality!*—I thanked them for taking such great care of us. The knot in my chest loosened. Baby steps.

~

Right around Christmas, after my hormones had leveled out and I'd pulled off the last of the surgical tape, my son discovered his jolly, effervescent laugh. His giggles rang through the silence like a choir of hand bells. My heart swelled as I hung his first stocking above the fireplace. Somewhere up in heaven my grandmother got her wings.

The snow never stopped falling that winter, and I never stopped nursing. In my former life, the clipped gray days of winter made me claustrophobic. As the mother of a newborn, I barely noticed the early sunsets or low skies. I nursed on demand all day and all night, every one or two hours, through cracked nipples. All the research suggested that when done properly, nursing should be convenient and painless. For me it was excruciating. The pediatrician suggested supplementing with formula when my son's weight gain slowed. Instead, I nursed more often and then pumped in between feedings, never letting a drop of formula touch his lips. My body was designed to nourish an infant completely, and I was willing to do everything possible to make breastfeeding happen. I was on a mission. Failure was not an option this time.

I joined several breastfeeding support groups on Facebook so I could troubleshoot on my phone while I nursed, never wasting a minute or a drop of the liquid gold. I learned that breast milk is a natural remedy for all kinds of physical ailments—eczema, diaper rash, cracked nipples, clogged tear ducts, and acne. But as my nipples healed and my son began to gain weight, I discovered the healing powers of breast milk went beyond skin deep. My body was finally getting it right; breast milk was soothing my soul. Every so often I'd massage a few drops into my incision scar because I figured it couldn't hurt. My husband told me I was a good mom. I started to think he might be right.

By the time the frozen ground yielded to purple crocuses, my son was sitting up on his own. He was a joyful little man. My everything. Even though my scar had begun to fade, every so often my caesarean would send me a little twinge, after a sneeze or during a yoga pose, as a gentle reminder that I was still in the weeds. Still, a sharp pain low in my belly was nothing compared with the neurosis I'd dealt with the first few months after my son's birth. There were even days when, with a breeze to my back and the spring sun warming my face, I would have said I was over it. That is, of course, if anyone had asked.

Breastfeeding had become natural. Nursing discreetly in public was no problem at all, and it no longer felt like my son was sucking hot magma through my nipples. I had everything a new mother could want—the cleavage of an unassuming porn star and an exclusively breastfed baby with chunky thighs. Even though I'd become a breastfeeding goddess, I still subscribed to the support groups on Facebook, and every so often, I felt shame for being a C-section mother in a breast-is-best world.

It always started with a disclaimer: THIS ARTICLE IS BEING SHARED TO PROVIDE MOTHERS WITH NEW INFORMATION REGARDING SURGICAL BIRTH AND SHOULD NOT BE VIEWED AS JUDGING MOTHERS WHOSE BABIES WERE NOT BORN VAGINALLY. Then came an article with only a tenuous connection to breastfeeding and then, in the comments, an all-out brawl. This was my introduction to the mommy wars, which I've discovered are fought with cheap shots and rarely face-to-face. As soon as a brave woman shared the circumstances of her caesarean, another three women, beneath cloaks of Internet anonymity, swarmed in with comments about how caesareans could be prevented if women trusted their bodies, ignored their medical providers, and birthed their babies at home in inflatable pools.

It always ended poorly, but I could never resist a juicy article detailing the physical and emotional trauma a baby experienced with delayed skin-to-skin contact or the long-term impact of a caesarean on a baby's gut flora and immune system. Then I'd scan the comments to see what the masses had to say about the C-section monsters that day. Read, scan, bleed. Repeat.

One summer evening, scrolling through Facebook on my phone, in an effort to stay awake until my son's first night feeding, I came across the headline: CAESAREAN SECTION MAY CAUSE EPIGENETIC CHANGES. The opening paragraph detailed the potential long-term impact of caesarean birth, including an increased risk of asthma, type 1-diabetes, obesity, and celiac disease. An angry ball of fire caught deep in my belly, replacing the usual self-deprecating burn. *What about all of us C-section moms following this group for breastfeeding support? Are we just supposed to read this article and consider ourselves lucky to have the information as we hug our imminently obese, diabetic children and clip coupons for gluten free animal crackers, and, you know, hope we have better luck next time?* I'm not sure if it was a generous pour of wine that evening or the culmination of 235 days with no more than three consecutive hours of sleep, but I refused to read the rest of the article.

Instead, I pecked out a declaration that *I* was refusing to read the article and encouraged other mothers in the throes of healing from surgical births to also surrender from the wars they were waging against themselves. I posted it to the comments, then walked absently into my bathroom and distracted myself from the article by taking out some frustration on what was left of my tooth enamel. After two minutes of aggressive scrubbing I looked back at my phone, which was lit up with a notification that I'd received a text from a lifelong friend. This friend is, on a typical day, as relaxed as I am after two shots of tequila and infinitely wiser. She'd given birth via caesarean four years earlier.

Shortly after her son was born her marriage ended, and, when the universe decided she needed to fine-tune her sense of humor, the doctors discovered cancer in her thyroid. In the text, she told me she'd read the article and said I shouldn't worry about it because the group of babies tested was so small (twelve!) that it was impossible for the doctors to draw any type of real conclusion; also, the study was Swedish and could not be trusted. Her words struck a chord. Rather than telling me I shouldn't feel bad about my C-section, she'd responded with logic and rationality, something this post-caesarean version of myself was incapable of doing. At this point, there was only so much I could continue to blame on my hormones. I was a thorough researcher, a careful analyst and, somewhere deep beneath my sleep-deprived crust, a woman capable of drawing independent conclusions. My friend made me realize that support groups would always share information; that other mothers would always have a better way; and that the word caesarean would always leave me achy and empty if I didn't come to terms with my birth experience. I decided to call a truce with myself—no more articles.

~

When I stopped picking at the scab long enough for it to heal, I could untangle myself from the complex web of guilt, shame, and regret my caesarean had helped me to spin. But beneath all that stick-to-your-fingers, messy stuff I still had plain old, uncomplicated sadness in my heart. I was disappointed that my first encounter with my son hadn't been the way I'd imagined it. The skin-to-skin bonding I expected had been replaced with a stiff, formal introduction. My son was swaddled in a blanket when the nurse presented him to me, his eyes slick with gel and his thick dark hair hidden beneath a white cotton cap. I'd been able to only pat his head politely before the nurse escorted him and my husband to the nursery so the doctor could put me back together again.

Nearly a year later, I looked back at the photos the nurse anesthetist took for my husband and me in the operating room that day. I was in search of the perfect photo to include on my son's first birthday party invitations. When I'd looked at these images in the past, I fixated on the tubes in my nose, the IV piercing my hand, the bonnet covering my hair, the microscopic gap between my front teeth, everything against a blue surgical backdrop. This time, I embraced my photos, viewing them from a renewed perspective. This time, I focused on the baby. Instead of seeing a red-faced stranger, I saw the boy I'd soothed, rocked, nurtured, and loved for the better part of a year. I recognized the furrowed brow that accompanied his forceful cry, his round belly and miniature clown's feet. A year later, I was no longer the woman who'd failed to deliver a baby the right way, looking at photographic evidence of her catastrophic error; I was a mother looking at photos of the day her life changed forever. I was looking at my son.

I thought I would cry when my son turned a year old, his first birthday some magical reckoning when I could physically release my final bit of sorrow. I'd imagined the tears streaming down my cheeks on the morning of his party, dripping into peaks of homemade vanilla icing I'd blend in my mixing bowl. Then, in a perfectly symbolic close to the first year of our lives together, my son would smash his cake—made with organic flour and his mother's love and tears—in front of his party guests. On the day of his party my tears never came, but I did manage to make him a gorgeous, wholesome cake. He recoiled in disgust when I tried to give him a taste of the icing, disappointing everyone who'd anticipated an adorably messy photo opportunity. I could only laugh when I later saw the photo of my son's snarl. He looked just like me.

The tears came more than two months later. I was sitting in a pew toward the front of a hundred-year-old chapel, wearing lipstick and a real bra for the first time in I couldn't remember how long. My husband, looking sharp in a black tuxedo, was at the altar with his dear friend, the groom. I watched the groom's sister wrestle with her toddler, a delicious, overtired cupcake of satin ruffles that matched the bridesmaids' gowns, while the congregation stood to welcome the bride down the aisle. Then the groom's sister read a short passage, which seemed to be, as if by divine orchestration, channeled from the heavens into the shadowy part of my spirit, and I cried. I thought of my son, who at that moment was at home with my mother, probably sloshing soapy water over the side of the tub and refusing to have his teeth brushed. That night, after the bride and groom shared their first dance as husband and wife, my husband and I shared our first dance as mother and father.

There's an old saying, that the moment a child is born, the mother is also born. It's a romantic notion that would look beautiful engraved into a silver photo frame, but it couldn't be more wrong. The seed that blossomed into this vibrant realization was planted in my heart that day at the wedding, when the groom's sister read this passage from *The Velveteen Rabbit*:

> "Real isn't how you are made," said the Skin Horse. "It's a thing that happens to you. When a child loves you for a long, long time [. . .] then you become Real.
>
> "Does it hurt?" asked the Rabbit.
>
> "Sometimes," said the Skin Horse, for he was always truthful. "When you are Real you don't mind being hurt."
>
> "Does it happen all at once [. . .]," he asked, "or bit by bit?"
>
> "It doesn't happen all at once," said the Skin Horse. "You become. It takes a long time."

After a very real year these words were the key to my understanding this simple truth: Mothers are not made. A woman is not made a mother in a hospital bed or on an operating table, or in a makeshift whirlpool, or a cab stuck in rush hour traffic. Motherhood is something that happens to a woman, not all at once, but with each lullaby and goodnight kiss. And it takes a long time. A woman becomes a mother rocking her child in the middle of the night and pumping breast milk during a conference call, tiny fingers wrapped around hers and a heavy body resting in her lap. She becomes a mother eating a cold dinner at the kitchen counter or waiting beneath the fluorescent lights at the pediatrician's office. A woman becomes a mother not in the wake of the grandeur of her child's birth, but during the accumulation of the small moments of adoration and the short, explosive moments of aggravation.

It took me just over a year to fully understand that my son's birth was not a test I needed to pass. It was not something I needed to do a certain way in order to become a worthy mother, not something to be defended or explained away, not something I had to prove to anyone, or to myself. It took a long time, but as the depths of my heart stretched beyond comprehension, I was able to let go of my caesarean and accept the heartache that came with it as part of motherhood. I didn't give birth just the way I'd planned, but my first day as a mother taught me that, even when all of my expectations go up in flames, absolute perfection can still rise up from the ashes. If I'm ever so blessed to become someone else's mother, I will know exactly what to expect. I will expect it to be frustrating, mind-blowing, and, at times, to hurt like hell. But as it happens to me all over again, I will feel exactly as I do this at very moment: chronically exhausted and eternally grateful.

the evidence

∽ *Lisa Solod* ∽

I HAVE A VERTICAL SCAR that travels from right below my belly button to well into my pubic hair, evidence of a child, then another, both unnaturally born: the trauma of, first, an emergency C-section by a doctor who was terribly nervous to the point of panic, and slit me stem to stern, and a second, scheduled C-section for my daughter. My scar is the only vertical one I have seen or known about, and for a long time, it felt like a major invasion. It was wide and long and fiery red. For months, with each stoop to lift my son, I felt the pull and pain of that scar. Thirty years later, it still itches occasionally. I rub it, and my babies' births come back to me.

In the mid-eighties, doctors were in short supply in the small Southern university town I found myself living in after my marriage. There was only one ob-gyn, a paternalistic older man who, when I expressed my desire to start trying for a baby, insisted I go on a series of hormones that made me so sick I could not get out of bed. I had, of course, informed him of my complicated gynecological history, which had involved, since my teens, misdiagnoses and numerous tests, laparoscopic surgery to remove cysts on my ovaries, and a multitude of doctors telling me that I would never have children. But he insisted on medication from the beginning. When I told him that the meds he wanted to prescribe to regulate my periods had, in the past, made me so sick I could not get out of bed, he grew angry with me for questioning him. He was gruff and unyielding and treated me as though I were stupid. I couldn't trust him. I was worried.

And then, by incredible chance, I was pregnant, three months after going off birth control pills. I went into a sort of shock. It couldn't be. I hadn't thought I would be able to conceive. I had been drinking wine and coffee, smoking cigarettes and pot. Yet I wanted babies. I would now have one. I quit smoking, gave up shellfish and fish with mercury, artificial sweeteners, soda, anything that might be the tiniest bit harmful. I walked, read books, took the requisite classes. I breathed and packed a suitcase. I was going to do everything by the book from that moment on, and I was going to have a child the natural way.

Nearly a trimester in, I needed to find a doctor quickly, and one I could trust. I found an experienced doctor who specialized in late-life and potentially complicated pregnancies. The problem was, he practiced in the university hospital, an hour and fifteen minutes away over a foggy mountain.

The appointments usually took up most of the day. At first, they were a chance to get out of town, go into the city, and do some shopping. I know I never imagined what it might be like to tackle that mountain in labor. All I focused on was that I had found a doctor who listened, instead of lectured. The truth was I was a little bit in love with him: he was from New Orleans and a bachelor, and he had a deep, gravelly Sam Elliott–kind of voice that put me at ease. In his waiting room sat girls as young as fourteen, grossly obese women, and many women older than I. I was thirty-one. My husband had a weird chromosome that ran in his family— though its effect was not known—so it was advised we have testing for that, as well as either amniocentesis or Chorionic Villae Sampling (CVS, in 1987, was a more modern equivalent). I chose CVS as it was done weeks earlier than amnio, and I wanted to know if anything was wrong with my child before the quickening.

Everything was normal. I was relaxed as I could be. Still, I felt enormous. I stupidly cut off all my hair and couldn't look at myself in the mirror: My hair had always been a source of pride. I was nauseated and could not eat cooked food for five months. I spent two days in the hospital with round ligament pain and feared I might lose the child. But the biggest worry was that I obsessed for much of the last three months of my pregnancy about the *first* three months, when I had imbibed alcohol, caffeine, cigarettes, and pot. Had I done something dangerous to my boy? At each visit Dr. Sam Elliott reassured me all would be well. Toward the end, even with the sleepless nights and the chronic indigestion, even with the long weekly drives over the mountain, I began to anticipate having my son on the outside of my body, where I could finally see him.

~

The night my water broke, I had eaten a huge meal. It was late September; my due date, according to me, was the next day. Dr. Sam and I had argued about the due date for the past six months; according to him, I was due October 15. I ate spaghetti with meat sauce. It would be three days before I had another meal.

When I climbed into bed with a book, it was midnight and pouring: the Shenandoah Valley rains had begun. All I wanted was a good night's sleep against the backdrop of water rushing down the gutters. I leaned back into the pile of pillows that supported my aching back and then, suddenly, felt a puddle on the mattress. My contractions began coming six minutes apart. My husband got my suitcase and started the car.

We drove cautiously for a half hour up the mountain in the black rain, the windshield wipers running at full speed. Only a couple of years earlier, my husband had maneuvered a huge U-Haul towing a car over these same mountains. As a kind of mantra to keep away the pain from contractions, I began to count in my head all the times we had never had an accident. The contractions sped up.

"Turn around," I said. "I don't think we'll make it."

My husband pulled to the side of the road, hands shaking. "Are you kidding?"

I imagined what it would be like to drive this road in the sunshine. And then I could imagine nothing but having the baby as soon as possible, even though we were still more than an hour away from Dr. Sam and his voice and the beautiful birthing room.

"No," I said. "I really don't think we can make it."

I had read all the pregnancy books; I had taken the Lamaze classes. I was well prepared. But I wasn't. I felt no confidence in my knowledge, and I had no idea how long it would really be before my baby was born. I could only think that I did not want to, would not, have my child on the side of the road, in the middle of the night, in the pouring rain.

My husband slowly turned the car around. Less than an hour later, he dropped me at the emergency entrance to our local hospital. I panicked again. I had heard that in the past few months the old paternal ob-gyn was thinking of retiring and had hired a young woman into his practice. I wondered: Who would deliver my child? That doctor I had fired? Or the new doctor? Would either of them even treat me? Did the hospital administration know I had fired my doctor? I felt sure they did. Our town was tiny. No speck of gossip was lost. I dreaded the thought of a stranger delivering my child. With almost thirty years of hindsight,

I think I should have let my husband keep driving. I should have ridden out the storm and my anxiety.

I explained to the staff and then the nurses that my doctor was at another hospital and that I didn't think I had time to make it. I asked them to call for the woman doctor, an unknown to be sure, but at the least no one with whom I had a grudge. Yet.

I labored hard for six hours. I had had plenty of time to make it over the mountain, but no experience to base my courage on and so no courage. I have never felt such fear as I did during those hours laboring in a cold, green hospital room while I waited for a doctor, any doctor, to show up. I was convinced I was being punished for not choosing them for my birth, that they were making me wait as long as possible. What I remember most is feeling utterly helpless, as if everything I had planned for had been taken from me.

I labored. All my plans, my desires, my convictions were gone. I tried not to weep. I wept. The baby wouldn't come.

I kept asking for the doctor, only to be told that she was on her way. I was sure she would not be there in time. I labored. The contractions grew closer. I tried the breathing I had learned, but that went out the window.

More than six hours after my first contraction, the doctor showed up. She was young, round, and unsure. She touched me as though I were the first woman she had seen in labor. I wanted to scream. Instead, I wept harder.

Pushing, again and again, did nothing. The fetal monitor they had attached when I came in showed that he was in distress. His heart rate dropped. The doctor looked as panicked as I felt.

"Please," I said. "Take the baby."

The doctor decided to do an emergency caesarean, and my plans dissolved into one moment when all that mattered was both of us getting out of that hospital alive and healthy. I was terrified. I was grateful. I was resigned. I was a failure.

There was no time for an epidural, so I had a spinal. Suddenly everything from the neck down was numb. They wheeled me into an operating room, draped a white curtain in front of my breasts, and began to cut. I could feel the pressure of the doctor's hand on my belly and the child pulled from my body.

Instead of holding my hand, my husband made the unfortunate mistake of peering over the drape, and I saw him turn white and begin to sway. A nurse caught him before he fainted. Only then did I consider what it must look like below the curtain. Nothing like the movies, no child emerging screaming from the birth canal; instead, a long, bloody incision from which an equally blood-covered baby emerged. A baby they had to gently slap so he would cry.

I was sewn up with a row of gold-covered staples. Later, when I showed them to friends, they were aghast. I had thought they must be normal. I think now that they were no more normal than that long, long vertical cut. The staples were sharp and stood out a half inch from my belly; they made holding and nursing my child an excruciating challenge, when I finally got the chance. The actual birth may have been painless, but there was nothing painless about the next weeks.

The day of my son's birth, groggy from the drugs and missing a night's rest, disoriented and depressed, I slept soundly for hours, until the pediatrician on call came into my room, woke me up, and remonstrated me for not nursing my child. I had been paralyzed from the chest down for hours, and nursing hadn't been possible. He said that the nurses in maternity had given my son sugar water and that if I did not take him that moment my son would never nurse at my breast. I burst into tears. No one had woken me. No one had brought my son to me. Now, when they did, he had trouble latching, and I had trouble holding him against my wounded belly. My breasts were still slightly numb. The nurses tut-tutted and told me it was my fault that he had gotten used to the bottle first.

For the next two days, while I recovered, the nurses ignored me when I buzzed them to bring my baby. I had to slide out of bed, hold on to the wall, and make my way to the nurses' section in order to speak to them. And still my son had trouble latching on. And still the nurses insisted on bottle-feeding him formula because they seemed worried he would starve. When I tried to describe my treatment to my husband and friends, they acted as though I were mad. I felt as if I had slipped into a Kafka-esque nightmare. As tentative about motherhood and frightened as I was, I couldn't wait to go home.

Once home, everything changed. I put the baby in a playpen beside the den, and I slept on a small bed in the guest room since I could not walk up the stairs. Even though my scar was a wide red welt that itched intolerably, my son was a joy. A happy child who, once my able and loving mother-in-law, mother herself to five children, sat with me for hours helping, managed to latch on easily. I held my baby to my wounded womb and felt the pain of the contractions as my body tried to regain its shape. I stroked my son's perfect head as he hungrily nursed. The nightmare of his birth rattled around in my head, but I kept pushing it out as best I could, even as I felt the rollercoaster of my moods, buoyed by hormones, guilt, pain, and a sense, an overwhelming sense, that I had failed both of us.

A few weeks after his birth, I sat down at my desk and wrote a note to my real doctor, the specialist from over the mountain. I apologized for not having the confidence to get to him, for letting us both down, for the way in which I had had to give birth. It was a crazy letter, as close to the edge of madness as I would get for a long while, painful and nearly incoherent. Absurd. Now I am not sure who the woman was who wrote that letter or why she felt she had to make amends with a doctor. Maybe it was because my treatment had been so brutal, so out-of-body in so many ways, that I needed someone to understand just how hard I had tried. Nothing had gone as planned and, ultimately, I had been numbed, summarily cut, and my baby pulled from my body.

Dr. Sam called me a few days later. I had nothing to apologize for, he said. Things happen. I burst into tears and told him how awful the experience had been, how traumatic, how badly scarred I was. He told me it would be all right. The boy was fine. I would be, too.

Years passed, my son grew, and I did, too. Mothering came naturally, and my son flourished. Five years on, pregnant with my second child, a daughter, I sat in Dr. Sam's office as we scheduled the C-section for two weeks before her due date. There was no chance of a vaginal birth without complications. The inexperienced, panicked doctor had seen to that with a hasty vertical cut. My womb was fragile and compromised. My doctor told me he would excise the nearly two inches of scar tissue, still raised and visible on my belly, and, after he had delivered my daughter, would pull it tight over my weakened womb. He advised me to have no more children after this, and I understood and agreed. After he took my child, he would tie my tubes.

Then he peered over his half glasses and said, "I want no more talk of failure. None of this was your fault. We will work with the damage done. We will deliver a healthy child. And all will be fine. Yes?"

I agreed. I nodded. I understood then, that no matter how I wished to think differently, some things, many things were out of my control. They always would be. Nothing illuminates that fact better than becoming a mother. But some small part of me, some tiny wound, remains unhealed. The scar reminds me of this from time to time. Rubbed by the zipper of my blue jeans, it sometimes aches. I remember the awe and despair at feeling my son pulled from my womb as I lay there, paralyzed from the chest down, and became a mother. My scar is still visible. I see it every day, the evidence of my motherhood.

c-section blues, or the biopsychosocial model for perinatal mood disorder

~ *Misty Urban* ~

WHEN MY SON WAS twenty months old and our family's lives had finally settled into a predictable routine—regular work schedule for Dad, preschool for older sister, and part-time day care for the boy, leaving Mom time to work—a book titled *Overcoming Baby Blues* landed in my hands for review. Edited by professors and psychologists working with the Black Dog Institute in Australia, the book was advertised as "A Comprehensive Guide to Perinatal Depression" for health practitioners and mothers alike. *Finally*, I thought, *a real resource for the poor women who suffer this.* I imagined I would find a lot to praise. From my comfortable vantage point of having passed two sets of screenings, the prenatal risk check and the six-week postnatal evaluation, the spectrum of perinatal mood disorders was something that afflicted other women, other moms. They got sad. They didn't feel connected to their babies. They found it hard to function, had fantasies of running away.

Then the authors outlined their biopsychosocial model for identifying causes of perinatal mood disorder, and I was surprised to find myself reflected in their list. Biological risk factors include hormonal influences like a thyroid imbalance (check), long-acting hormone-based contraceptives (check), a caesarean section or traumatic delivery (check), and extreme fatigue or insomnia during the postnatal period. Double check with exclamation points.[1]

Psychological factors that presented a risk included temperament or personality styles exhibiting self-criticism, anxiety, perfectionism, and socially avoidant tendencies.[2] Four more checks for me. Of social stressors, the most significant included lack of sleep (yeah, but that's everybody) and lack of support, practical/instrumental or emotional.[3] Check and check again. Altogether, the results suggested a 100 percent chance that this mother would develop some form of postnatal depression (PND).

Then I read on and discovered that what is called PND can include acute anxiety and, sometimes, insomnia. I sat back and let the book fall closed. At last I knew what had happened to me. It had a name. It had a list of risk factors. I could have seen all this coming. Would it have helped, if I had been aware of this checklist in advance? Would it have improved my coping mechanisms if I'd known what I was up against? I might have appreciated having a label, but I suspect the black wave would have risen up and pulled me under, all the same.

I wouldn't say the C-Section was traumatic. "Traumatic" has been used by witnesses to describe the birth of my daughter, a vaginal delivery. Her beautiful head, when the OB finally pulled it out, measured fifteen-and-a-half inches in diameter. The average baby head, mind you, is between eleven and fourteen inches. The few people I told about my partial third-degree tear said, "A tear takes longer to heal than a C-Section." The vacuum left my daughter with a cephalohematoma (a big lump on the head) that caused a great deal of worry the first three months of her life. My daughter is four now, and I can still see the birthmark on her forehead from her struggle to emerge.

The second time around—with different doctors, in a different state—the ultrasound showed a biggie from the start. At thirty-six weeks, baby boy weighed in at an estimated nine pounds. Averaging a half-pound gain per week, he would emerge a hefty eleven-pound watermelon. Macrosomia (big baby syndrome) triggered a policy of my OB practice to "recommend" a C-section. Watermelon babies are at higher risk for labor complications, birth trauma, and stillbirth. Plus, I was an elderly bigravida—pregnant for the second time, and over thirty-five. We thirty-five-plus are a class all our own in obstetric circles, presenting a profile of special risks and problems that only worsen as our creaky reproductive apparatus continues to break down.

"I know it's not what you want to hear," the OB said, kindly putting his hand on my arm. "But no one here will do a vaginal delivery with a baby that size."

I was, to be honest, shocked. I thought that C-sections were A Taboo Topic in the maternity ward. The birth class for my first child had skipped the C-word entirely. The mountains of pregnancy literature I'd read hinted that a C-section was an affront to motherhood and humanity. Women who gave birth "naturally" glistened through their labor, bonded better with their infants (all that oxytocin, you know), and enjoyed the quiet superiority of having fully participated in the ancient rite of birth. Mothers who had C-sections were at higher risk for postpartum complications. Their recovery times were slower. They felt robbed of a "real" birth experience. They grieved.

When I mentioned I was carrying a future NFL linebacker, the nurse who gave me the tour of the birth facility told me she'd seen a woman deliver a thirteen-pounder. "She worked that squat bar like a pro," she said.

But I wasn't being offered the chance to show off my birthing chops. I walked to the parking lot and sat in my car, trembling. I hadn't had any enchanting, soft-focused visions about my delivery. My birth plan consisted of "emerge with healthy baby." What rocked me was having the decision taken out of my hands. My authority over my own body had been yanked away, overridden by sets of statistics that had little to say to my particular experience. I'd already signed the form saying I didn't want an epidural. A C-section hadn't even been on my radar, and now I had to prepare for one. Maybe there *is* a grieving process, I thought, and then I burst into tears.

But in the end, what mattered most was the health and safety of the little fetal pig. In the competition for worst-ever childbirth stories, I already had a runner-up trophy thanks to my daughter, the third-degree tear, and the stitches that permanently changed my nether landscape. At least I would spare my son vacuum extraction and birthmarks that never faded. From the parking lot, I called the office to schedule my C-section on their recommended day, in thirty-nine weeks. There was an upside; now I could give my parents a firm date for when to come down for the birth.

I went into labor in the wee hours of Easter morning, a week before my scheduled delivery. The day before, we celebrated our daughter's second birthday, and I thought the uneasiness in my stomach was from too many fried wontons. The Easter baskets were sitting where I hid them when we bundled our daughter into the car and drove to the hospital in the next town, bringing the hospital bag, the diaper bag, and her nap blanket.

The sole nurse on duty when they rolled my wheelchair into the maternal ward at 4:00 AM was a woman I'd met at a social event for my Mothers of Preschoolers group. I wished it were someone I didn't know checking my cervix. After an hour of tests and another hour of observation, I heard the calls going out from the nurse's station, dragging a whole crew of people from their beds, their families, their church service. "So we're going ahead with the C-section," my doctor said, appearing at my bedside in his scrubs and shower cap. Even though baby boy had already wriggled his way into the birth canal, they were going to pull him out by his feet.

It was now 6:30 in the morning. I'd had no sleep. My husband wouldn't be present for the birth because we knew no one in this town who could take our daughter. A nurse offered to snap pictures with my camera, which seemed unspeakably pitiful. I was told they would take the baby directly to the nursery to evaluate him; I wouldn't get to hold him until everyone else on the floor had prodded and poked him first. And I was getting an unscheduled C-section, red alert, top of the list of Things Not in the Birth Plan. I went for levity.

"Care to give me a C-tuck?" I asked my OB.

He smiled. He didn't look tired. "I'll give you a bikini incision," he said. "In a year, you won't even be able to see it."

There were seven people in the operating room, and two of them were there just to support me by touching my arms and narrating events behind the blue curtain. That was nice. It took two attempts to get the anesthesia needle placed correctly. I'm not fond of needles, even when they're pouring warm numbness into my central nervous system. I lay back and became the body on the table, following instructions, waiting for the doctors to do the work that should have been mine.

My slick, squalling super baby weighed in at nine pounds one ounce. I heard the numbers called out over the screaming. *You made me get a C-section*, I thought, *and he's nine pounds, one ounce*. The squalling continued, and after some discussion the baby nurse wiped him down, wrapped him up, and put him on me. The only available skin was my shoulder, since the doc was stitching me up. My boy turned his nose toward my neck, and the screaming stopped. The oxytocin came in floods.

They removed him for a brief stint under the warming lamp while I was moved and cleaned up and outfitted in my non-embolism socks, but my Easter egg was nested in my arms by the time my husband returned from McDonald's, which, with its indoor playground, was the logical place to amuse a two-year-old at 7:00 Sunday morning. I recovered on schedule. Baby pooped, got his inoculations, latched and fed. I was on track to win the Best Patient Ever Award because I was so cheerful and cooperative, and asked for nothing, except when I developed a sore neck shortly after they removed the morphine drip. The celebratory pictures show me draped in a hot towel as if I've just emerged from the locker room after a tough game. For a week, my neck was locked into the forward position and my spine was so stiff I had to sleep in a chair. I suggested it was a reaction to the anesthesia; surely having a foreign substance introduced into your spinal fluid could have this effect? The hospital nurses all said, "These maternity beds are really uncomfortable. Everyone says so."

Baby Boy was perfect, not a single mark on him, unless you count the enormous cephalohematoma he developed from the time spent burrowed into my pelvis. It swelled up one side of his head, leaving him lopsided. We called it his horn—he was half angel, half devil. The blood reabsorbed around six weeks, the same time I passed my postnatal depression questionnaire without raising a blip. I was in such a fog of sleeplessness, painkillers, and constant activity that I had no idea how I was feeling and answered the questions mostly by guess. I didn't have time to think about my

feelings. My husband, deciding we needed the income more than
I needed his help, went back to work after one week. My parents
stayed a bit longer. I got through the days of aching body,
potty-training a two-year-old, and lugging around a hefty newborn by asking myself one question: Which of these billion things
requiring my attention needs to be dealt with *now*?

Turns out, if anyone's asking, a caesarean incision doesn't heal
any faster than a vaginal tear. At least not when you're elderly.

While the authors of *Overcoming Baby Blues* agree that C-sections
are a risk factor for developing perinatal depression, not all
research supports this. In the Obstetrics and Gynecology section
of the *International Scholarly Research Notices*, an abstract titled "Postpartum Depression: Is Mode of Delivery a Risk Factor?" claims
that vaginal birth, elective caesarean section, or emergency caesarean section had no effect on EPDS [Edinburgh postnatal
depression scale] scores for the women in their study. Interestingly,
the research subjects who had experienced excessive vomiting
during their pregnancy, had a history of depression, or were
housewives earned significantly higher EPDS scores. The authors
concluded that "healthcare providers should be aware of postpartum depression risk in nonworking women . . . and apply the
EPDS to them for early detection."[4]

Nothing in my conversations with my doctors, at any point in
my pregnancy or post-delivery management, covered my working
situation. When my daughter was born, we'd lived in Idaho, where
I taught English at a small college. I had six weeks of family leave,
the summer to bond and recuperate, and a wonderful daycare that
took her the days my husband was working. Then my husband
accepted a job in central Illinois. We both wanted to live closer to
our friends and family in the Midwest, and I had the starry-eyed
idea that I would write full-time. Even when I learned, a whole

month after our move, that I was pregnant again, I decided I could still make time to write. That summer, I researched a conference paper in the mornings while my daughter played and napped in the hotel room, and we spent the afternoons exploring our new town. Shortly after we bought and moved into our new house, I found a lovely facility that would take our daughter part-time while I went to the coffee shop, sipped decaf mochas, and drafted novels. Then my Easter egg hatched and my journey to the Underworld began.

Somewhere in the postpartum haze, I ran across the information that the hormones get stronger with successive pregnancies, and I thought, *So that's what's happening to me.* For baby one, I had been an A+ gestating student. For baby two, I gained too much weight, craved fatty foods, had intense ligament pain, and showed a nine-month profile at twenty-four weeks. Not only did I have no memory but I started forgetting words with such frequency that I feared early onset dementia.

None of this improved once the sprout was out. Baby Boy, allowed to nuzzle my neck during those first crucial moments, decided he never wanted to be out of physical contact, ever. He liked nursing and did it often. He wanted to be held when he slept. He wouldn't have let me leave him anywhere, even if daycare were still within the family budget which, with two kids, it was not. As the days disappeared into the endlessly recycling activities of grooming, feeding, supervising, and maintaining a moderately clean living environment for two small beings with incessant demands, everything I enjoyed sank further on the priority list. There was no time to write, and no energy for it during the rare moments both kids were sleeping. Since we were in a new place, I knew no one nearby who I could call to take the kids for half an hour so I could shower, read, take a walk, do yoga, any of the things that kept me in the realm of the sane people. The friendships made at my moms' group were still new, too fragile to lean on. My parents and closest friends lived six and seven hours away. I had no back-up, no bolt-hole. No village.

And then I stopped sleeping.

At first it was a funny joke: Baby's sleeping through the night, but I'm not. I would wake thinking I heard him cry and then lie awake for hours, mind trotting on a hamster wheel of self-accusatory, fearful, or simply mundane thoughts. Very soon it was no longer funny. I tried to use the hours I was awake. I journaled a lot; I read. But most of those hours were a dark haze of feeling too tired to do anything, yet too wired to rest, body burning with exhaustion while the mind circled in its airless and predictable loops. I lurked through the house with earplugs and pillow, trying to find rest in the guest room, on the couch. The time-sickness that clutched at me during the day disappeared with the darkness.

When I saw my doctor to get my thyroid evaluated, I told him I was losing sleep. He simply pointed to my two kids, crowded into the office with me. At the follow-up to get the results of my blood test, when I hinted again that I still wasn't sleeping well, he said, "You know, those hormones can stay in your blood for a year."

I didn't understand what he meant. In my defense, my brain was functioning in basic survival mode, mostly from the middle and back portions; the prefrontal parts with their essential cognitive functions were starving, unable to do their necessary repair work during sleep. I spent my extended waking hours researching sleep remedies. I tried nighttime teas, hot baths with salts or lavender oil. Antihistamines ramped me up instead of tamping me down, so most over-the-counter sleep aids were out of the question. Herbal remedies like melatonin or Hyland's Calms Forté were like popping sugar pills, great taste, not so filling. I tried guided meditation and delta beats. The first worked sometimes;

the second, weirdly, made me more anxious and tense, my altogether unplastic brain resisting the manipulation.

I thought my symptoms were the problem. That sudden whole-body spasm jolting me awake: That, I learned, is called a sleep start. That heart-pounding sensation of falling off the top of a building, opening your panicked eyes to feel yourself drilled into the bed: Also a sleep start, sometimes called a hypnic jerk. Waking up convinced I had heard a door slam somewhere, that had a more fun name: exploding head syndrome. I thought about enrolling in a sleep study. I read about fatal familial insomnia and joked to my husband, at least I don't have *that*. But I did have acute, chronic insomnia, which in prolonged cases can lead to hallucinations and paranoia, not to mention physical illness. Something was haywire in my brain and no one could tell me what it was.

On the upside, the days following what I logged in my sleep journal as "red nights"—a grand total of one hour of sleep, maybe two, which by the time my son was nine months was two or three times a week—I spent in a hazy cocoon. I was less reactive, slower to annoy, less subject to bouts of sudden, blistering rage. I wondered if in some way the insomnia was an adaptive strategy, my body trying to help me survive this period of being alone in the house every day with a stubborn two-year-old and a clingy infant. But I had lost my resilience and sense of humor. I had exhausted all my resources and was burning up the reserves.

When the red nights increased to three and four a week, I went to my doctor with sleep journal in hand. The insomnia was getting "pretty bad," I said, with that feminine instinct to minimalize. He focused on the anxiety. I didn't see the connection; I'd been prey to anxiety all my life, could usually pass for normal with the help of yoga, journaling, and gainful employment. He referred me to the psychiatry office and prescribed clonazepam, a benzodiazepine used to treat seizures. I looked it up on my phone while the kids played in the bath. Clonazepam is classified by the American Academy of Pediatrics as class D, a drug known to cause risks in pregnancy, and there was no data showing it safe for breastfeeding. Desperate as I was, I wasn't going to take the chance I could harm my son. Back I went to the doctor's office and embarrassed both him and me by bursting into tears. I wasn't just asking for help; I was begging. "I have to be able to take care of my kids," I bawled, Kleenex crumpled in my fist.

"All right," he said, "we'll bring the hammer down." He prescribed Ambien and called the local counseling center with a referral.

The Ambien didn't help my insomnia. But the therapy did.

My journey didn't end with an epiphany in the counselor's office, but she helped lay down a trail of crumbs. She helped me step back from the whirling thoughts and harness the wild monkey mind. She didn't blame me that I missed my work and wanted to be writing. Find the time, she said. Find daycare, find the money, make it happen. She didn't let me wallow; she made me focus on the next step that would get me out of the morass.

I started exercising. This initially involved twenty minutes of hollering at the kids to stay away from the moving bars of the elliptical machine, but it helped. I used the Ambien nights before a talk, a deadline, or on family visits. I weaned my son and went away to a medieval conference that made me feel like a scholar again. Every couple of weeks, when I felt that tightness under the skin that meant the rage monster wanted to surface, I cut a little yellow pill in half and took the clonazepam. It drew a sweetly fuzzy purple outline between me and the abrasive world.

Slowly, the light changed. Slowly, I came back to myself. And slowly, if not as fast as I would have wished, my sleep improved.

For all the research on pregnancy and childbirth that I had done for baby #1, for all the information I had reviewed for baby #2, nothing about my experience registered as PND until that blessed baby blues book floated, by an editorial whim, into my hands. I thought depression meant, you know, depression. I hadn't known that increased anxiety could come in that shopping cart, or that my thyroid history might put me at risk. It now seems obvious to me that, with no chance of being heard or heeded during the day's incessant clamor, my body started screaming for help at night. If I had simply flagged the insomnia as a sign of postnatal anxiety, I might have been able to save myself six months of torture that has probably shortened my life and most certainly did not result in class-A caretaking.

Or, maybe it wasn't really PND. I was never diagnosed, never evaluated. Maybe I was just really, really stressed out. Maybe things just hit me harder because of my age, because I was less elastic, because pre-baby two I had been established in a career I now deeply missed. Maybe the drugs did help. Or maybe the hormones finally flushed, the way my neck loosened after the anesthetic worked its way out of my system. With my daughter, despite the curdling stories I now tell about her birth, my body got to follow its biological blueprint of expelling the baby through the designated channel. My son and his placenta got pulled out, not pushed, and who knows what biochemical signal got interrupted and was left floating around the bloodstream, confusing and annoying everything else. The C-section delivered my boy to me safe and whole, and I will always be grateful for that. But I simply don't believe the medical studies that claim a caesarean doesn't increase the risk for PND. My own experience says otherwise, and I'll bet I'm not alone in this.

Then again, I'm beginning to think that what we call postnatal depression isn't really an anomaly so much as a matter of where a

mother falls on the spectrum of What Happens to Your Hormonal
Body After You Give Birth. I suspect that somewhere between the
80 percent of new mothers who experience passing baby blues and
the 13 percent who are diagnosed with PND lies a great mass of us
who don't know, can't articulate, or don't want to admit what is
happening to us for fear of being grouped under the Something Is
Wrong With You umbrella, with its attendant emotions of shame
and guilt. We, along with our partners, our care providers, and
our support networks, need to recognize that we are standing in a
hugely overwhelming moving ocean of motherhood, subject to
changing tides and waves. Sometimes we feel a tug around the
ankles, maybe on bad days a slap around the knees. Sometimes we
float too far out of our depth and get sucked under by a riptide,
where we end up fighting to keep our nose above water and some
air in our lungs.

I'm not suggesting we minimize PND, which in its severest
form can manifest as postnatal psychotic depression or puerperal
psychosis. We've all read the horror stories about moms harming
themselves or their babies while in the grip of this agony. Instead,
I'm suggesting we stop thinking of PND as a special seating area
and recognize that any of us wander, at various times, in and out
of the Inability to Function foyer. There's no shame in it. It's the
cost, and a perpetual risk, of entering this wondrous and often
alien land of motherhood.

More than anything, I think our cultural conversation needs
to reflect the reality that childbirth is a gigantic challenge and it's
not all snuggling adorable talcum-scented baby skin or jokes about
pee, puke, poop, and needing a glass of wine. There is a shadow
side that needs to be acknowledged. Sometimes, the chubby little
arms around your neck are not a wreath but a stranglehold; sometimes the writing in the sand is not "I love you" but "Help." Just
as our collective adulation of the gestating body creates more

wounds for the women who would desperately love to birth their own baby and have been denied that chance, our cultural reverence of the Mother glosses over the high price women pay for their bundles of love, in everything from permanent marks on the body to spiritual dark nights of the soul. The costs of pregnancy and motherhood to a woman's physical, emotional, and mental well-being are rarely reckoned with in the broader public conversation, and, if glanced at, are expected to be cheerfully paid as fees for the Sacred Honor of Nourishing Life.

I'm not asking for a Purple Heart. I am just glad to see the beginnings of more frankness, more freedom in the conversations about the mothering experience. It's not one big long serotonin high for everybody. We make sacrifices. We emerge with scars.

Like my C-scar. Two years later, the caterpillar wriggling across my lower belly is as livid and red as ever. It itches often. More than once I have been caught, in public, trying to slip a hand down the waistband of my pants for a scratch. Another one of those things no one tells you.

along those lines

∾ *Susan Hoffmann* ∽

I CAN'T SEE the jagged line—the surgical scar—but I know it's there. I know the path it took, and where it began.

I was living in Minneapolis in the summer of 1980, finishing up grad school in art history at the University of Minnesota. My boyfriend Michael, a professor in engineering, had just landed the academic job of his dreams, a faculty position at the California Institute of Technology in Pasadena. We were preparing for our wedding and our move out West when my GP, during a routine check-up, felt an abdominal mass.

"We should talk," he said, concern in his voice. "My nurse will show you to my office after you've dressed."

The nurse quietly led me to a small office next to the examining room, where I sat for what seemed like an eternity. What was wrong?

"Sorry for the wait," he said, "but I wanted to consult with a colleague." And then he explained his concern. He'd discovered a mass—a large one—and worried it might be a malignant uterine tumor. "My colleague and I both agree that you need surgery immediately, given the size and the rapid rate of growth of the mass."

Within days, I met with a gynecological surgeon, who ordered an ultrasound. The imagery showed an enlarged uterus, but not the exact position of the mass. It was either inside the uterus, or lodged in the wall, he told me. To learn the location and determine whether it was cancer required surgery, my only option.

"You may need a hysterectomy," he told me, "in case the tumor's malignant." He described the process. "I'll make a vertical incision, belly button down." His voice still rings in my memory, animated and eager, as he summed up his plan. "A nice cut will give me elbow room in case I need to clean you out."

Even as fear sent my mind spinning—Was it cancer? Would I die? If I survived, without a uterus, would my boyfriend reconsider our marriage? I knew this surgeon would not touch my body, would not have the chance to "clean me out," like a dusty closet full of clothes I didn't need. I asked for another doctor.

When I met with the next surgeon, a few days later, I immediately felt at ease. He was Dutch and spoke English with a charming lilt, an odd memory, certainly, but one that reminds me how his calm presentation helped me trust his advice. Like his colleague, he recommended a vertical incision, cutting first through the abdominal muscles and then into the uterus. He would try to save the uterus, he reassured me, should I want children. In truth, children weren't foremost in my mind. I wanted to survive the surgery, whole. Michael and I hadn't talked about having a family. We both had our hearts set on our careers. But what if we did want children? Shouldn't I find a way to preserve that option?

I scheduled the surgery, a myomectomy. The surgeon spent two long hours removing a large, gourd-sized fibroid tumor lodged in the wall of the uterus. Luckily, it was benign. He did have to make a long incision, "belly button down," but was able to carefully hull out the tumor by making only a very small incision in the wall itself. Maybe he told me, after the surgery, that I could have children, but only with a C-Section. I can't remember.

I do remember the painful recovery. I stayed in the hospital for nearly a week, on the Labor and Delivery floor. Turning from one side to another caused a sharp, needle-like pain to radiate across my stomach. The pain became worse the more I rested, like an expanding balloon pushing in all directions and causing pain with each sharp nudge. A nurse finally told me, with a smile, "It's gas! This always happens when they open the stomach. Get up and walk around. You'll be fine." Michael teased me into walking down to the nursery. "They put your tumor in a jar, right next to the babies!" Of course, they hadn't, but the joke got me out of bed.

The day I was discharged, the attending nurse explained the regimen to follow at home: take the antibiotics as prescribed, keep the incision area clean—no bathing, and don't lift anything heavy. "Imagine a gallon of milk," she said. "Nothing heavier than that or you might cause the incision to tear." Otherwise, I was fine for the wedding, and fine for our move. The incisions would heal, both on the surface and deep within. In years to come, and unknown to me at the time, another surgeon would cut along the scarred skin to deliver our children. But that summer in Minneapolis, my dreams focused on the future and our adventure out West, where my husband and I would pursue our careers under the warm California sun.

~

I started a freelance business, writing educational materials and teaching for Los Angeles art museums. Michael settled into his faculty life at Caltech. Carefree and happy, we bought a small house in Pasadena, and then a crazy Labrador retriever, and, a few months later, a second. Somehow, getting those dogs seemed to be our way of becoming a family. When our friends talked about pregnancies and babies, we shared stories of the pups. Children of our own? Not part of our plan—not until the winter of 1981, when family tragedy struck.

My sister called. "Daddy didn't make it," she said. "He was in the ambulance when his heart stopped." He'd been sick, but his recovery seemed to be progressing well. He was so young—still in his fifties. Stunned, I flew home. We buried Daddy alongside his family in a tiny cemetery in rural Missouri, where he had grown up. His father lay in a grave nearby, as did his only brother, a childhood victim, in 1923, of diphtheria. I remember my grandmother that day, stoic but devastated at her loss. "It's not right for a mother to bury her children," she kept repeating. "It's not right." We stood there on that cold November day, the week before Thanksgiving, the gray sky heavy with our sadness. It wasn't right. None of it.

When I returned to Pasadena, grief overwhelmed me. I turned down work and retreated to the safety of our house. The few times I ventured out, to pick up groceries or run errands, I became angry, as if the people around me—the ones smiling and laughing—didn't know the world was different, now that my father was dead. My mother brought Grandma out for New Year's, thinking a trip to sunny Southern California to see the Rose Parade might brighten all our moods. No such luck. One night before dinner, we watched in horror as Grandma stumbled down a hallway and slumped over from a stroke.

How much grief could my family bear? Mother flew back to Kansas. She had her own life to put in order, with Daddy's death. Grandma was admitted to a Pasadena hospital for her recovery and rehab. In the midst of it all, over these many weeks, I was pregnant without knowing it. When I did realize I'd missed my period, the doctor estimated conception two weeks after my father's death. "Women often become fertile after a death in the family," he told me. I took comfort in this idea, that life could follow death. It seemed like a light, piercing what seemed to be a very dark cloud hanging over me.

After the doctor's visit, I went to the hospital to see Grandma. She lay still in her bed, not yet strong enough to sit or stand. I pulled a chair close to her bed. "I have some great news!" I told her. She smiled and squeezed my hand. This was her sign of affection, this little squeeze. It reminded me of the many times in my childhood she'd taken my hand to share a little joke, or soothe an injury. "Remember the shots," she said faintly, her eyes moist with tears. She never spoke of the little boy she lost, all those years ago, to diphtheria. But she never hesitated, nor had my grandfather, to remind new parents to vaccinate their children. What she didn't say, but what I heard, was that repeated phrase at Daddy's burial, "It's not right for a mother to bury her child."

Looking back on that spring of 1982, when my pregnancy and my grandmother's illness overlapped, both unfolding in the grief of Daddy's death, I recognize how the extremes of joy and sadness held hands as tightly as we did that afternoon at the hospital. I think, too, or want to imagine, that Grandma and I found strength in each other. She did recover, and boarded a plane back to Kansas. And my pregnancy progressed normally. But it wouldn't be typical. The tragedies my family had endured that winter would influence the choices I had to make.

"We need to talk about a C-section," the doctor told me at one of my first exams. He had reviewed my medical record and explained his recommendation to schedule a C-section well before the onset of labor. "The surgeon made a long vertical incision for your myomectomy," he said. "I'll have to follow that same line, and use a general anesthesia."

"Can't you make a small horizontal cut?" I asked, thinking about what we called a "bikini line," a less invasive way to perform a C-section. No. He explained crisscrossing the abdomen with horizontal and vertical cuts would further weaken the uterine wall. "The myomectomy incision has made a natural birth dangerous." If I knew this, I hadn't fully understood the nature of the danger. "During labor, the wall might break, killing the baby and sending you into shock. You'd have to be at the hospital within an hour to save your life." I remember he told me the odds of this happening—only a two-percent chance. As I write this today, those odds seem incredibly small. But, at the time, I wasn't in the mood to gamble. With Daddy's death and Grandma's stroke, and her words, playing on a loop in my mind, "It's not right for a mother to bury her children," I didn't hesitate to take his advice.

My husband and I shared our pregnancy experience with our friends, some with young children, others beginning families. We talked about finances and schools and names. We shared notes on doctors and hospitals. When the discussion—at parties, over lunch, during walks with the dogs—turned to Lamaze and natural childbirth, Michael would joke that we didn't have to think about any of that. "Check in, check out with a baby!" he'd say, adding, "Maybe they'll put in a zipper this time, you know, for easy access to babies and tumors!"

Our humor, born in the fear of what lay ahead, and memories of the myomectomy scare, puzzled our friends. When we detailed the surgery I'd had and would have to repeat, one that required a general anesthesia, they wondered how Michael felt being barred from the delivery room. We tried to explain how we had no choice—and we had none, nor do parents today—in witnessing surgery, *any* surgery, performed under a general. Someone would inevitably bring up the need to immediately bond with the newborn, a romantic notion thought to guarantee a well-adjusted child. We have no choice, we would say, we have no choice. On the ride home from a party, after hearing these questions yet again, Michael said, "Why would a husband want to see a surgeon take a knife to his wife?"

We retreated to the perimeters of these pregnancy conversations, settling into our own private zone of humor. We laughed at the serious nature of choosing baby names, at books that listed names most apt to assure success for children—best schools, best jobs. We came up with an alternate list, one listing made-up names that honored Los Angeles. A front-runner was the nicely alliterative "Hollywood Freeway Hoffmann." Another choice was 110 North Hoffmann, to honor the freeway we'd take home from the hospital.

As the due date approached, humor didn't mask the anxiety over the surgery that lay ahead. My blood pressure soared, sending me to the Labor and Delivery floor for observation, where a team of doctors rushed into their own version of panic. They would stabilize me, send me home, and I'd return the next day. This went on for a week until I approached the scheduled date for delivery.

The day I delivered, the C-section went smoothly. I woke up in the recovery room to see my husband smiling as he told me the news, a boy, healthy and strong. We named him Hobie, after the inventor of a small sailboat my husband used, growing up along Lake Michigan. (Yes, we kept the transportation theme.) An orderly wheeled me, still hooked up to monitors and IVs, to my room, where I had my first chance to hold my baby. He moved in my arms like a swimmer, back and forth, like he was riding a wave. It was a motion I enjoyed when he was still in the womb. I hadn't seen him delivered, but I knew he was mine, ours.

I also knew, remembering my recovery from the myomectomy, that I had to get up and walk, no matter how much it hurt. After the nurse took Hobie to the nursery, Michael helped me up for a walk down the hospital hallway. I felt much stronger than I had after the myomectomy. Maybe this was due to the C-section being relatively fast, keeping me under the general anesthesia for minutes instead of hours. Just as likely, I was euphoric after a successful delivery and surgical procedure. But I couldn't celebrate my new motherhood completely, not quite yet. There were a few more days in the hospital, and an unexpected surprise the very next day.

"Time for blood work," a technician announced as he swept into my room before dawn, pulling back the privacy curtain that separated my bed from the door. A nurse followed soon after, listing the activities for the day, as I watched blood being drawn from my arm.

"After you finish breakfast, we'll bring the baby to you," the nurse said. "And then, after his feeding and return to the nursery, you'll attend a meeting for the C-section moms." She looked up from her notes and shrugged her head toward the door. "You'll see the room, just across the hall." She left before I could ask any questions. Was the meeting about caring for our babies, or ourselves; about what to expect in recovery? I was ready, I thought, all set to contribute what I knew: Get up and walk.

At the appointed time, I walked over to the meeting room. I felt good and looked forward to sharing upbeat stories about our babies and our recovery. About a dozen mothers had gathered, all, like me, wearing hospital-assigned robes. Long faces and vacant stares met me as I took a seat. Before I could start up a conversation, a man entered the room and opened the session. I can't remember if he was a doctor, a nurse, or a therapist, only that he spoke in a serious, somber voice.

"We know you're depressed," he said. "We know you feel horrible that you weren't able to have a natural childbirth. This is normal. Most women feel this way." He droned on as I looked around in disbelief. Some of the mothers were nodding their heads in agreement; others wiped away tears. We had all had live births, I thought. We were mothers. Wasn't this the goal?

Apparently not. We were supposed to feel guilty, diminished as women, angry with the medical establishment. We were led to believe that we would be, or might believe ourselves to be, bad mothers because of the C-section. The facilitator rattled on with a list of reasons we should feel as badly as we did. But I didn't feel badly. Not about the guilt he presumed we shared. I felt horrible for the women, though, who sat there, crestfallen, burdened by cultural ideas on the perfect birth they hadn't had.

I still share that memory with young friends who are pregnant. "Don't feel bad if you have to have a C-section," I tell them. "Remember the goal is the baby. A C-section is just a medical procedure, not a mark of failure or, worse, a condemnation of your choice of delivery method."

~

Four years later, in 1986, we prepared for the delivery of our second child, also a planned C-section. We would use the same hospital, the same doctor, and follow the same program, which involved a general anesthesia. My husband would wait outside the delivery room, as was required, and await the news from the doctor. "It's a boy," he told Michael, who then told me, in the recovery room, "a boy, nearly eleven pounds!" When I first held him, I felt every ounce of that weight, and, as he nursed aggressively, I imagined the boy he would become, big and ravenous.

Michael drove home to take care of our older son Hobie. I settled into a room, ready to steal some much-needed rest. I was surprised when a nurse wheeled the baby in and set the crib at the end of the bed.

"Won't he be in the nursery?" I asked.

"Of course not!" she said. "All babies stay with their mothers now. It's required. Babies need to bond with their mothers." I protested, pointing out that I'd just had a C-section, with a long abdominal incision that made it difficult to sit and stand, that I wasn't supposed to lift anything heavy—like a giant baby—that might cause the incision to tear. How could I stand up and lift the baby for nursing?

"You'll need to do it when you get home, so you'd better start now." And she marched out of the room.

The baby wailed in his crib. Was it really safe for me to lift him? I pressed the call button for the nurse. "Can't you please wheel him to the nursery so I can rest up from surgery?" She came into the room, irritated. "You need to bond with your baby! You have to learn how to take care of him!"

Bewildered (and exhausted), I struggled to sit, then stand, and slowly walk to the crib. I gave my little boy a kiss and pushed the crib to the door before slowly heading back to bed. Since my room was next to the nurses' station, his loud cries caught their attention. The nurse returned. I made my same request. And she pushed him out the door and down to the nursery. I fell asleep.

I awoke to the voice of a doctor, someone I'd never met. He stood at the end of my bed, clipboard in hand. "Are you having trouble with bonding, experiencing some dislike of your baby we need to discuss?" He glared at me over the top of his glasses. "The nurse tells me you don't want the baby in your room." I explained again that I was recovering from a C-section and only wanted a brief time to regain my strength before going home. He gave me a terse lecture on maternal bonding and how studies showed that immediate bonding, preferably through seamless gestation and vaginal delivery, created the healthiest, best-adjusted babies.

So here was the new guilt gift for C-section moms, I thought. No vaginal delivery equals maladjusted babies. It seemed bizarre (and does still) that, on the one hand, the medical establishment should recommend a C-section, and then, after birth, another camp of this same team could fault me for following that advice. I didn't respond to the doctor's lecture. He noted something on my chart and left the room without another word.

My husband brought me and the baby home a couple of days later. We settled into our new family life. It wasn't until my first check-up with my ob-gyn that I faced a new, unforeseen problem.

We started the visit cordially. He had been my doctor for nearly five years, had seen me through both C-sections. We often began my appointments catching up. Yes, I told him, the baby was fine and our older son, too. "And you?" he said. Feeling stronger by the day, I said. Then his expression changed, and his tone, too.

"There's a problem," he said. "You heal badly. The scarring along the incisions I've made, and the one from the other surgery, have left a thick rope of a line along the uterine wall. It was hard to stitch you up. You shouldn't have any more babies."

I slumped in the chair at his desk. I remember looking away, not wanting to believe what he was saying. He had moved to a new facility and into a lovely office, with high ceilings and floor-to-ceiling windows. The glorious California sun glowed its golden warmth that afternoon. But, in my memory, all I felt was a sickening claustrophobia of being confined by scars I couldn't see. The marks of my surgeries, the evidence of medicine removing a tumor and delivering my boys, these lines had morphed into a barrier I couldn't cross.

"You probably shouldn't have had this one," he continued. I could tell from his voice, which became softer, more deliberate, that this prognosis was hard for him to deliver. "The uterine wall won't survive another pregnancy. It would break, killing you and the baby."

I left the appointment terrified. I went to the car and drove home, hearing the same questions loop around in my mind. What if our birth control failed and I did get pregnant? How could I justify ending one life to save my own?

Michael tried to soften the impact of the doctor's news. "Maybe we should have had that zipper put in," he joked. But humor didn't work this time. We grew cautious, sexually. We didn't want another pregnancy and the risks it carried. We had our family, our two sons. We would protect what we had.

⁓

The boys are grown now. I rarely consider their lives in terms of their C-section births. I do think about my scars—the thick rope of a line the doctor described. They are hidden reminders of the surgeries I needed and the obstacles I faced in their aftermath. But now, all these years later, I also know that my motherhood began along those lines. And the path they've followed, as I raised my family, have been my lines to draw.

Acknowledgments

WE ARE INDEBTED to a large and generous community. It took several years to bring this book to fruition, and the editors thank our families, friends, and colleagues who supported us along the way. We thank the brilliant, honest, and creative essayists who believed in the importance of this collection, trusted us with their work, graciously accepted feedback, and stuck with us through a journey that was, at times, uncertain. We thank Kathleen Glasgow for her invaluable insights as she helped us shepherd the manuscript through its first three years as well as her continuing encouragement.

We thank our agent, Jennifer Thompson, for her powerful belief in this book and deft navigation of the publishing world. We also thank everyone at Nordlyset Literary Agency for championing the collection. We thank our editor, Batya Rosenblum, for her unwavering support with this project, as well as the whole team at The Experiment. We are grateful to Maggie Smith for thoughtfully reading this collection and writing a beautiful Foreword.

We also want to thank writing colleagues and friends who generously shared our call for submissions, connected us with essayists, and offered valuable feedback. Our gratitude goes to Lauren Alleyne, Victoria Blanco, Gabrielle Civil, Jennifer Kwon Dobbs, Mackenzie Epping, Laura Flynn, Jennifer Bowen Hicks, Steve Horwitz, Kathryn Kysar, Sheila O'Connor, Angela Pelster, Robin

Schoenthaler, Amy Shearn, Julie Stevenson, and Theresa Wenzke Schroeder.

Finally, Amanda is grateful for the steadfast support and love of James Austin and their daughter, Fiona. She thanks Rachel Moritz for an inspired and thoughtful collaboration. Rachel sends her gratitude to Amanda Fields and her love and appreciation to her partner Juliet Patterson and their son, Finn.

Permissions Acknowledgments

An earlier version of "Upside Down" by Mary Pan first appeared online as part of the EPIC Writers 2017 Contest.

Images in Nicole Cooley's essay, "Notes from the Lying-In Hospital," are sourced from the National Library of Medicine at the National Institutes of Health. Italicized text is from "Cesarean Section—A Brief History," by Jane Eliot Sewel, National Institute of Health, U.S. National Library of Medicine, nlm.nih.gov/exhibition/cesarean/index.html.

An excerpt from Nicole Cooley's poem "Rampion," first appeared in her book, *The Poets Grimm* (Story Line Press, 2007) and is reprinted here by permission of the author.

Notes

INTRODUCTION

1. McCulluch, Sam. "Highest C-Section Rates by Country." *Bellybelly. com*. bellybelly.com.au/birth/highest-c-section-rates-by-country/.

2. smith, s. e. "Trans? Good Luck Accessing Reproductive Health Care." *Rewire News*. rewire.news/article/2016/05/17/trans -reproductive-health-care. See also Martin, Nina. "Black Mothers Keep Dying After Giving Birth and Shalon Irving's Story Explains Why." *NPR News*. npr.org/2017/12/07/568948782/black-mothers -keep-dying-after-giving-birth-shalon-irvings-story-explains-why.

3. Morris, Theresa, *Cut It Out: The C-Section Epidemic in America* (New York: New York University Press, 2013), 16.

PART TWO, INTRODUCTION

1. Sewell, Jane Eliot. "Cesarean Section—A Brief History." National Institute of Health, US National Library of Medicine. nlm.nih.gov/ exhibition/cesarean/index.html.

2. Plenda, Melanie. "Once a C-Section, Always a C-Section?" *The Atlantic*. theatlantic.com/health/archive/2014/05/ once-a-c-section-always-a-c-section/362088/.

3. Morris, Theresa, *Cut It Out: The C-Section Epidemic in America*, 7.

4. Thiekling, Megan. "Sky-high C-section rates in the US don't translate to better birth outcomes." *STAT.* statnews.com/2015/12/01/cesarean-section-childbirth.

5. Morris, Theresa, *Cut It Out: The C-Section Epidemic in America*, 5.

6. Wesley, Erika. "Cesarean Delivery on Maternal Request." The American College of Obstetricians and Gynecologists. acog.org/Clinical-Guidance-and-Publications/Committee-Opinions/Committee-on-Obstetric-Practice/Cesarean-Delivery-on-Maternal-Request#2.

7. Morris, Theresa, *Cut It Out: The C-Section Epidemic in America*, 12.

THE EMPEROR'S CUT

1. Gannon, Megan. "Prehistoric Grave May Be Earliest Example of Death During Childbirth." LiveScience. livescience.com/49680-siberia-grave-mother-twins.html.

2. Conis, Elena. "Cesarean section's ancient history." *Los Angeles Times.* articles.latimes.com/2006/may/01/health/he-esoterical. See also Sewell, Jane Eliot. "Cesarean Section—A Brief History." National Institute of Health, US National Library of Medicine. nlm.nih.gov/exhibition/cesarean/index.html.

3. van Dongen, Pieter W. J. "Caesarean section—etymology and early history." *SAJOG.* August 2009, Vol. 15, No.2. sajog.org.za/index.php/SAJOG/article/view/158/117.

4. Betrán, Ana Pilar. "The Increasing Trend in Caesarean Section Rates: Global, Regional and National Estimates: 1990–2014." *PLOS One.* journals.plos.org/plosone/article?id=10.1371/journal.pone.0148343.

5. Boatin, Adeline Adwoa, et al. "Within countries inequalities in caesarean section rates: observational study of 72 low and middle income countries." *thebmj.* bmj.com/content/360/bmj.k55.

6. World Health Organization. "World Health Organization Statement on Caesarean Section Rates." who.int/reproductivehealth/publications/maternal_perinatal_health/cs-statement/en.

7. Betrán, Ana Pilar. "The Increasing Trend in Caesarean Section Rates: Global, Regional and National Estimates: 1990–2014." *PLOS One.* journals.plos.org/plosone/article?id=10.1371/journal.pone.0148343.

PART THREE, INTRODUCTION

1. Ellison, Katherine, and Nina Martin. "Nearly Dying in Childbirth: Why Preventable Complications Are Growing in US." *National Public Radio.* npr.org/2017/12/22/572298802/nearly-dying-in-childbirth-why-preventable-complications-are-growing-in-u-s.

C-SECTION BLUES, OR THE BIOPSYCHOSOCIAL MODEL FOR PERINATAL MOOD DISORDER

1. Parker, Gordon, Kerrie Eyers, and Philip Boyce, *Overcoming Baby Blues: A Comprehensive Guide to Perinatal Depression* (London: Allen & Unwin, 2014), 34.

2. Parker, Eyers, and Boyce, *Overcoming Baby Blues*, 40.

3. Parker, Eyers, and Boyce, *Overcoming Baby Blues*, 49.

4. Goker, Asli, et al. "Postpartum Depression: Is Mode of Delivery a Risk Factor?" *ISRN Obstetrics and Gynecology.* hindawi.com/journals/isrn/2012/616759.

About the Contributors

JUDY BATALION was born in Montreal, studied at Harvard, and worked as a curator and comedian in London before settling in New York City. She was a columnist for *The New York Times*'s Motherlode, and her essays about parenting, relationships, religion, and health have appeared in *The New York Times, Vogue, Washington Post, Jerusalem Post, Salon, Forward, Tablet, Cosmo,* and many others. Her first book, *White Walls: A Memoir About Motherhood, Daughterhood, and The Mess In Between,* was shortlisted for the Vine Award for Canadian Jewish Literature, longlisted for the Leacock Award for Literary Humor, and optioned by Warner Brothers, for whom Judy is currently developing the TV pilot, *Cluttered.* Judy's second book, about Jewish women who fought in the resistance against the Nazis, will be published in 2020. *Daughters of the Resistance* has been optioned by Steven Spielberg's Amblin Partners, and will be published across Europe and in Brazil and Israel. Find her at judybatalion.com

SARA BATES is a former lawyer who unearthed her love for creative writing after becoming a stay-at-home mom. As an aspiring novelist, Sara steals writing time in the predawn hours and whenever she can find a babysitter. Writing about the C-section experience healed and strengthened Sara, and she went on to deliver her daughter via VBAC in 2016. She lives outside of Philadelphia with her husband and two children. You can find Sara on Instagram: @embracemypace.

TYRESE L. COLEMAN is the author of the collection *How to Sit*, a
2019 PEN Open Book Award finalist, published in 2018. Writer,
wife, mother, and writing instructor, she is an editor at *SmokeLong
Quarterly*, an online journal dedicated to flash fiction. Her essays and
stories have appeared in several publications, including *Black Warrior
Review*, *Buzzfeed*, *Literary Hub*, The Rumpus, and *Kenyon Review*. She is
an alumni of the Writing Program at Johns Hopkins University and
a Kimbilio Fiction Fellow. Find her at tyresecoleman.com and on
Twitter at @tylachelleco.

NICOLE COOLEY is the author of seven books, most recently the
two collections of poems *Girl after Girl after Girl* and *Of Marriage*. She has
received the Walt Whitman Award from the Academy of American
Poets, the Emily Dickinson Award from the Poetry Society of America,
and a National Endowment for the Arts Grant. Her work has appeared
in *The Atlantic*, The Rumpus, *Paris Review*, *Poetry*, *American Poet*, and
Callaloo, among other journals. She directs the MFA program in
creative writing and literary translation at Queens College, City
University of New York, where she is a professor of English. She lives
outside of New York City, with her husband and two daughters.

JEN FITZGERALD is a poet, essayist, photographer, and native New
Yorker who received her MFA in poetry at Lesley University and her
BA in writing at the College of Staten Island (CUNY). She teaches
creative writing workshops online and around New York City. Her first
collection of poetry, *The Art of Work*, was published in 2016. Her essays,
poetry, and photography have appeared in such outlets as *PBS
Newshour*, *Boston Review*, *Tin House*, and *New England Review*, among
others. She is living in and restoring a 200-year-old hotel/boarding
house on Staten Island as she completes her memoir.

CAMERON DEZEN HAMMON is a writer and musician whose work has appeared in *Ecotone,* The Rumpus, *The Literary Review, The Butter,* Brevity's Nonfiction Blog, *Houston Chronicle, Columbia Poetry Review,* and elsewhere. Her essay "Infirmary Music" was named a notable entry in *The Best American Essays 2017,* and she is a contributor to *The Kiss: Intimacies from Writers.* Her music can be found on iTunes and Spotify and has been featured on Houston Public Media's KUHF, Houston Pacifica Radio's KPFT, as well as the PBS television shows *Skyline Sessions* and *Oxford Sounds.* Cameron is the host of *The Ish* podcast, and her first book, *This Is My Body: A Memoir of Religious and Romantic Obsession,* is forthcoming.

SUSAN HOFFMANN's work has been published by *Literary Mama, Persimmon Tree, Gravel, 500 Pens,* and in the anthology *Nature's Healing Spirit.* Her essay "A Boy Like Mine" was a finalist in the Tenth Glass Woman Prize. Retired from her career in art museum education, and a writer and lecturer on art history, Hoffmann lives in Los Angeles and writes personal essays inspired by her family. She blogs about her grandfather's World War I experience using letters he sent home at ww1betweenthelines.com. Her two sons were delivered by C-section in 1982 and 1986.

LATOYA JORDAN is a writer from Brooklyn, New York. She is the author of the poetry chapbook *Thick-Skinned Sugar.* She has an essay listed as "notable" in *Best American Essays 2016,* and her writing has appeared in *Mom Egg Review, Poets & Writers,* The Rumpus, *Mobius: The Journal of Social Change,* and more. LaToya received an MFA in creative writing from Antioch University Los Angeles. She is mother to an amazing kid and wife to an English teacher. Visit her at latoyajordan.com.

DANIELA MONTOYA-BARTHELEMY is a queer Xicana from a small town in northern New Mexico. Her business, Mama Sin Vergüenza, was born out of her first son's birth and her passion for sexual health and social justice. The services offered reflect her gifts in balancing strategic health research with holistic modalities of care. Daniela aims to support individuals navigating the life and death cycles around reproduction and trauma transmutation. She loves getting into the nitty-gritty academics of public health research and enhancing that knowledge through intuition. In addition, she is slowly integrating Mexican Traditional Medicine and somatic psychology practices into her services as she learns more from trusted teachers.

CATHERINE NEWMAN is the author of the memoirs *Catastrophic Happiness* and *Waiting for Birdy*, the middle-grade novel *One Mixed-Up Night*, and the kids' craft book *Stitch Camp*, which she coauthored with Nicole Blum. She also writes the blog Ben and Birdy and the etiquette column at *Real Simple* magazine, and is a regular contributor to many publications. She lives in Amherst, Massachusetts with her family.

AIMEE NEZHUKUMATATHIL is professor of English in the University of Mississippi's MFA program. Her newest collection of poems, *Oceanic*, was published in 2018. She is also the author of the forthcoming book of illustrated nature essays, *World of Wonder*, and three previous poetry collections: *Lucky Fish*, *At the Drive-In Volcano*, and *Miracle Fruit*. Her most recent chapbook is *Lace & Pyrite*, a collaboration of nature poems with the poet Ross Gay. She is the poetry editor of *Orion* magazine and has published in *American Poetry Review*, *New England Review*, *Poetry*, *Tin House*, and has twice appeared in the *Best American Poetry* anthology. Honors include a poetry fellowship from the National Endowment for the Arts and the Pushcart Prize.

ELIZABETH NOLL is an editor at the University of Michigan. She earned an MFA in creative writing at the University of Minnesota and has worked as an archaeologist and journalist. She lives in Ann Arbor with her husband and son and two cats: Bella and Groot.

MARY PAN is a writer and family medicine physician with training in global health and narrative medicine. Her work has been published in *Intima, Hektoen International, Till, Blood and Thunder,* and elsewhere. She lives in Seattle with her husband and three young children. More at marypanwriter.com.

SOOJIN PATE is a writer and educator who is dedicated to praxis that centers the lives and experiences of historically marginalized peoples. Since receiving her PhD in American studies, she has taught courses on self-care, critical race theory, women of color feminism, and US history and literature at various colleges and universities in the Twin Cities. She is the author of *From Orphan to Adoptee: U.S. Empire and Genealogies of Korean Adoption,* and *Motherloss: A Memoir* (forthcoming). Her writings on self-care, self-love, African American literature, and Korean adoption have appeared in various journals and edited volumes.

ALICIA JO RABINS is a writer, composer, performer, and Torah teacher. Her first poetry book, *Divinity School,* won the 2015 American Poetry Review/Honickman First Book Prize, and her second, *Fruit Geode,* was published in 2018. Alicia is the creator of *Girls in Trouble,* an indie-folk song cycle about the complicated lives of women in Torah, and *A Kaddish for Bernie Madoff,* a one-woman chamber-rock opera about the intersection of finance and spirituality. Find her at aliciajo.com.

ROBIN SCHOENTHALER, MD, is a Boston-based cancer doctor, mother of two young adult sons, essayist, and storyteller. She writes about her experiences as a physician, a solo parent, and general observer of life issues at the extremes. Her essays have appeared in *Boston Globe, New England Journal of Medicine, Readers' Digest, Brain, Child* magazine, *Pulse* magazine, *Boston Globe* magazine, and many others. She is a Moth GrandSLAM contestant and a two-time Pushcart Nominee. Read more about her work at DrRobin.org.

MAGGIE SMITH is the author of, most recently, *The Well Speaks of Its Own Poison* and *Good Bones*, from which the title poem was called the "Official Poem of 2016" by Public Radio International and has been translated into nearly a dozen languages. Smith's poems have appeared in *The New York Times, Tin House, The Believer, Paris Review, Kenyon Review, Best American Poetry,* and on the CBS primetime drama *Madam Secretary.* A Pushcart Prize winner, Smith has received fellowships and awards from the National Endowment for the Arts, the Academy of American Poets, the Ohio Arts Council, and the Sustainable Arts Foundation.

LISA SOLOD is a widely published essayist, journalist, and short story writer whose work has taken honorable mentions in *Zoetrope, New Millennium* (twice), and *Meridian Magazine*, among others, as well as a notable citation in *Best American Essays 2013.* Her work has appeared in *The New York Times, Washington Post, International Herald Tribune, Boston Globe, Boston Herald, Boston* magazine, *Brain, Child,* Huffington Post, *Dame, Purple Clover, The Mani-Festation,* and *Lilith,* as well as almost two dozen literary magazines and anthologies. Her novel, *Shivah,* out for submission, was a finalist in the Autumn House fiction contest in 2015, and a semifinalist in the William Faulkner– William Wisdom fiction competition in 2017, where her short story "Salt" was a finalist. She is the author/editor of *Desire: Women Write About Wanting.*

About the Editors

AMANDA FIELDS is an assistant professor of English and the Writing Center director at Central Connecticut State University. She has published creative work in *Indiana Review, Brevity, So to Speak, Nashville Review,* and others. She coedited *Toward, Around, and Away from Tahrir: Tracking Emerging Expressions of Egyptian Identity,* and has published scholarship in *Kairos: A Journal of Rhetoric, Technology, and Pedagogy; Journal of Adolescent Research; Sexuality Research and Social Policy;* and edited collections. Among her honors is the 2016 *Kairos* Best Webtext Award. She holds a PhD in rhetoric and composition from the University of Arizona and an MFA in creative nonfiction from the University of Minnesota. Learn more at amandajfields.com or on Twitter at @aj_fields.

RACHEL MORITZ is the author of the poetry collections *Sweet Velocity* and *Borrowed Wave,* which was a finalist for the National Poetry Series and the 2015 Minnesota Book Award in poetry. Her work has appeared in *American Letters and Commentary, Colorado Review, Iowa Review, Tupelo Quarterly, Water-Stone Review,* and other journals. Among her awards are grants from the Jerome Foundation and the Minnesota State Arts Board. Rachel lives with her partner and son in Minneapolis where she works as a teaching artist and content developer for museum projects. More at rachelmoritz.com.

JACINDA TOWNSEND is the author of *Saint Monkey*, which is set in 1950s eastern Kentucky and won the Janet Heidinger Kafka Prize and the James Fenimore Cooper Prize for historical fiction. *Saint Monkey* was also the 2015 Honor Book of the Black Caucus of the American Library Association, longlisted for the Flaherty-Dunnan First Novel Prize, and shortlisted for the Crook's Corner Book Prize. Jacinda received her MFA from the Iowa Writers' Workshop and went on to spend a year as a Fulbright fellow in Côte d'Ivoire. She recently finished a novel called *Kif*. Jacinda is mom to two children, about whom she writes frequently.

MISTY URBAN has published award-winning short fiction in several journals and anthologies, online and in print, and in two collections: *A Lesson in Manners*, winner of the Serena McDonald Kennedy Award, and *The Necessaries*. Her medieval scholarship focuses on medieval romance and monstrous women, including the coedited collection *The Footprint of Melusine: Tracing the Legacy of a Medieval Myth*. When not teaching writing at Muscatine Community College or working on her novel, she entertains herself by watching her two children play. Find her online at mistyurban.net or at femmeliterate.net, a website about feminism, literature, and women in/and/of books.